A COMPLETE BOOK OF
REIKI HEALING

A COMPLETE BOOK OF
REIKI HEALING

*Heal Yourself, Others,
and the World Around You*

BRIGITTE MÜLLER & HORST H. GÜNTHER

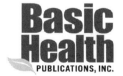

Basic Health
PUBLICATIONS, INC.

The treatments and results explained in this book are based on decades of experience. The healing power of Reiki has helped the authors as well as countless others. However, the authors and the publisher of this book remind you that a medical doctor may need to be consulted before treating an illness. Although Reiki flows freely, be aware that you carry the responsibility for how, when, and to whom you apply Reiki.

The publisher does not advocate the use of any particular healthcare protocol but believes the information in this book should be available to the public. The publisher and authors are not responsible for any adverse effects or consequences resulting from the use of the suggestions, preparations, or procedures discussed in this book. Should the reader have any questions concerning the appropriateness of any procedures or preparation mentioned, the authors and the publisher strongly suggest consulting a professional healthcare advisor.

Basic Health Publications, Inc.
28812 Top of the World Drive
Laguna Beach, CA 92651
949-715-7327 • www.basichealthpub.com

Library of Congress Cataloging-in-Publication Data is available through the Library of Congress.

Translated from the German by Teja Gerken and Brigitte Müller
Edited by Dixie Black Shipp
Editor, 2012 edition, Roberta W. Waddell
Photographs by Horst H. Günther, Germany
Illustrations by Atelier Duschl, Germany
Interior production: Gary A. Rosenberg
Cover design: Mike Stromberg

Printed in the United States of America

10   9   8   7   6   5   4   3   2   1

CONTENTS

ACKNOWLEDGMENTS

Our gratitude goes to the divine power of the universe, which enables us to transmit the gift of healing hands to this planet through Reiki initiations.

We also want to thank the following individuals: Dr. Mikao Usui, who after searching for many years, rediscovered Reiki; Dr. Chu-jiro Hayashi, and Mrs. Hawayo Takata; and especially Phyllis Lei Furumoto, who initiated both of us as Reiki Masters/Teachers.

We would also like to thank our parents and everyone who has supported us and Reiki in the past years through words and action.

Our universal gratitude extends to all our teachers, as well as our students, who have also been teachers; and all our Reiki friends who have shared their experiences with us.

In love and gratitude, we dedicate this book to
Dr. Mikao Usui
Dr. Chujiro Hayashi
Hawayo Takata
Phyllis Lei Furumoto
To the healing and harmony of this planet
with all its forms of life
To all those who are searching
And to all those who have received the gift of Reiki

1

WHAT IS REIKI?

R eiki is an ancient healing art, which channels universal life energy through the hands of a practitioner into the body of a receiver. Because it is a universal, God-given power, Reiki belongs to anybody who is ready to receive the gift of healing hands. Anyone, even children, can easily learn it, no special knowledge is needed except the initiation and transmission of power through a Reiki Master/Teacher.

Reiki is a Japanese word meaning universal life energy. The universe—the space around us—is filled with endless and inexhaustible energy. It is this universal, pristine, and productive source of power and energy that also keeps us alive. Reiki is this natural healing energy, and it flows through the hands of the Reiki channel in a powerful and concentrated form.

We are all born with this universal life energy, but as we go through life we become less open and the flow becomes less pure and free.

- *Rei* means universal life energy.

- *Ki* is a part of *Rei* and it flows through everything alive, including our own individual vital life energy.

- *Ki* is known to Christians as *light*, to the Chinese as *Chi*, to Hindus as *Prana*, and to Kahunas as *Mana*. It is also called *Bioplasma* or *Cosmic Energy*.

Reiki was rediscovered in Japan in the 19th century by a Christian monk named Dr. Mikao Usui, who found references to it in a 2500-year-old Sanskrit document written by one of Buddha's disciples. In the Usui System of Reiki, the healing energy is spontaneously and effortlessly transmitted from one's own body to another organism, through the touch of hands. The strength of the energy depends on the need of the receiver. Reiki goes through any kind of material, including clothing, plaster, bandages, or metal. The healer, being a channel, only transmits the universal life energy, no personal energy is taken from the healer; on the contrary, both giver and receiver are simultaneously strengthened and enriched with energy.

Anyone giving Reiki is more than just a channel; that person *becomes* Reiki and universal life energy. It is the God within who accomplishes this powerful task. It is not the ego; it is the *I AM* presence, the divine self through which the healing takes place. Self-healing energies are awakened through the transmission of Reiki because you can only heal yourself. Because of this, both the Reiki practitioner and the person receiving Reiki are experiencing *self-healing* during the treatment. Anyone seeking or wanting to give Reiki healing can become a channel. Reiki does not conflict with any religious or meditative practices or rituals; it will only enrich and strengthen their universality.

Reiki supports medical treatments, including such therapies as massages, foot reflexology, cosmetic massages, acupressure, acupuncture, chiropractic treatments, breath therapy, lymph drainages, or psychotherapy. It is effective wherever the hands of a practitioner touch a receiver because Reiki hands radiate healing energy at any time in any place. Because of this, Reiki is especially helpful to those in healing profession.

Reiki brings the body and mind into an even balance and works on all levels: the physical, spiritual, emotional, and soul level. Reiki encourages self-healing, strengthens body and soul, removes barriers or blockades, balances the chakras, rebuilds harmony, and flows in unlimited quantity. Through Reiki you will experience the blessing of spiritual growth and change. Reiki is the divine grace of God, an immeasurable gift.

The History of the Usui System of Reiki

Until this century, the history of Reiki was transmitted from teacher to student mainly through an oral tradition.

Dr. Mikao Usui, the founder of Reiki, lived in Kyoto, Japan toward the end of the nineteenth century and served as a Christian priest and leader of a small local university. At one of his Sunday services, a student asked if he took the word of the Bible literally. Usui affirmed that he did, but his student wasn't satisfied with the answer. He asked, "In the Bible it says that Jesus made the sick healthy, that he cured them, and that he walked on water. Do you believe that Jesus walked on water, simply because it is written? Have you ever experienced something like this yourself?" "No," said Usui, "I have never experienced such a thing. But I do have faith in the words of the Bible." The student replied, "Maybe this blind faith is enough for you, but I would like to see these things with my own eyes."

This dialogue brought a great change to Usui's life. The next day he quit his work and traveled to the United States to attend the University of Chicago. There he studied ancient Christian writings and received a doctorate in Ancient Languages. He was always trying to understand the secret of the healings by Jesus Christ and his disciples, but he was unable to find what he was looking for.

During his studies he had learned that Buddha also had the power to heal. He decided to return to Japan in search of further Buddhist

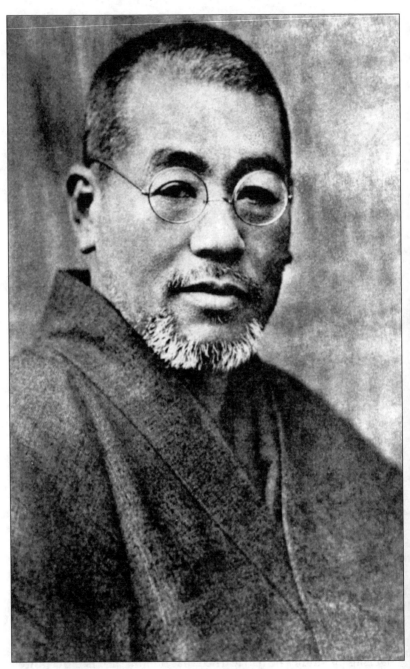

Dr. Mikao Usui

teachings. Back in his homeland, he traveled to many monasteries. This is how he finally met an older Abbot in a Zen monastery who was also interested in healing. He stayed in the monastery and began to search through the old Buddhist writings—the Sutras—for the key to healing. At first he studied the Japanese translations of the Sutras. Because he couldn't find an answer, he learned Chinese. But even in the Chinese translations of the Sutras he could not find any leads.

Usui did not give up. He learned Sanskrit so he could read the original Buddhist writings. Finally, in an ancient Sanskrit document written by an unknown disciple of the Buddha, he found the formula, the symbols, and the description of how Buddha healed that he had been seeking for seven years.

He had thus rediscovered the knowledge, but still lacked the power to heal. Following a consultation with the Abbot, he decided to go to a holy mountain in Japan to fast and meditate for twenty-one days. He placed twenty-one small rocks on the ground in front of him to serve as a calendar, removing one every day. During these days, he read the Sutras, sang, and meditated.

In the middle of the twenty-first day, it was still very dark when Dr. Usui finished his meditation and prayed fervently, "Father, please show me the light." Suddenly, moving rapidly toward him in the sky, he saw a bright light. It became bigger and bigger as it came toward him and hit the middle of his forehead, at the third eye. He fell to the ground, lost consciousness, and moved into a trancelike state of being. In this higher state of consciousness he saw many rainbow-colored bubbles: blue, turquoise, lavender, and pink. The symbols he had seen earlier in the Sanskrit Sutra appeared in front of him in golden letters as if they were on a giant screen.

This was the key to the healing powers of Buddha and Jesus. This enlightening experience marks the beginning of the Usui System of Reiki.

The sun was high in the sky when Usui regained consciousness. To his surprise, he was full of energy, and not exhausted or hungry

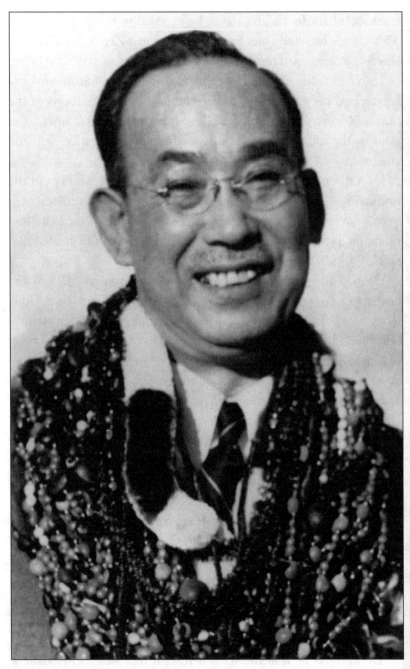

Dr. Chujiro Hayashi

as he had been the day before. On his way back to the monastery, Usui stumbled, injuring his big toe. When he held his hand over it, the bleeding stopped, and the pain went away.

Soon he found a hostel where he ordered a meal. While he waited, the innkeeper's daughter appeared with a swollen red cheek and a face in pain due to a toothache. Usui asked for permission to touch her face. He held both her cheeks in his hands, and within minutes the swelling went down and the pain went away. "You are no ordinary monk," said the very surprised girl.

Upon his return to the monastery, he learned that the Abbot was in bed with arthritis. After resting, Usui applied his healing hands and the Abbot's pain eased.

Several weeks later, Usui decided to go into the slums of Kyoto to heal the sick. He healed many there and sent everyone who was young and able out to look for work. After seven years of doing this had passed, he realized the same familiar faces were returning to the slums again and again, all with the same conditions they had when he had first found them.

He was very discouraged, and asked why they had come back. They told him they preferred to live as they previously had, and showed no gratitude for the life he had tried to help them live.

Usui was shattered, and realized that although he had healed the symptoms of illness in their bodies, he had not taught them a new way of life. This caused him to create the *Reiki Rules of Life. (From the journal of Hawayo Takata)*:

> *Just for today do not anger*
> *Just for today do not worry*
> *Honor your parents, teachers, and elders*
> *Earn your living honestly*
> *Show gratitude to every living thing.*

Given our many experiences and recent realizations about posi-

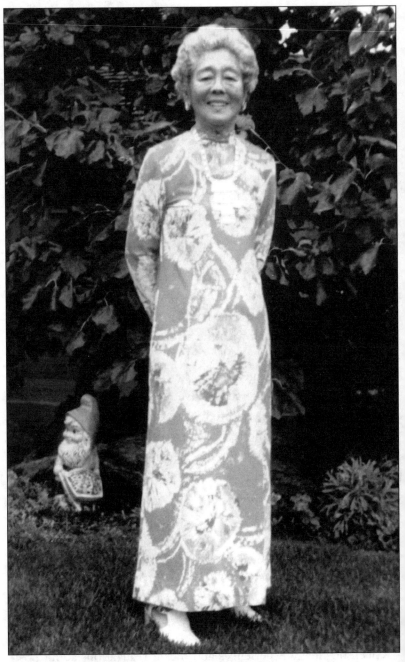

Mrs. Hawayo Takata

tive thinking, the authors have adapted these Rules of Life for today's age, and turned them into a more contemporary form.

Spiritual Rules of Life
Just for today
Be free and happy.
Just for today
have joy.
Just for today
you are taken care of
Live consciously in the moment.
Count your many blessings with gratitude
Honor your parents, teachers, and elders.
Earn your living honestly.
Love your neighbor as you love yourself
Show gratitude to all living things.

Usui left the slums of Kyoto and began to teach. He taught people to heal themselves and he passed on his rules of life so people could heal their minds as well as their bodies.

Dr. Chujiro Hayashi, a retired Marine Officer, wanted to serve humankind and became Usui's student. Initiated by Usui, Hayashi felt a deep vocation to practice Reiki and became Usui's closest assistant. As Usui got closer to the end of his life, he made Hayashi a Reiki Master and trusted him to keep and care for all the teachings.

Hayashi founded the Reiki Healing Clinic in Tokyo where Reiki was taught and used to treat people. From Hayashi's documents it is clear he believed that Reiki finds the cause of physical symptoms, which it then balances with the right vibrations (or fills with the needed energy), in order to reestablish health.

Hawayo Takata, a young woman from Hawaii, came to Japan in 1935 to have a tumor surgically removed, but just before the operation, she heard an inner voice telling her the procedure was not necessary and there was another way for her to be healed. After she

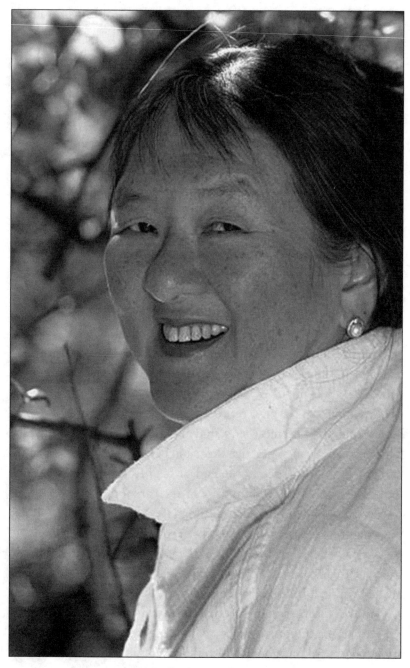

Phyllis Lei Furumoto

talked with the doctor, his nurse, Ms. Shimura, took her to Dr. Hayashi's Reiki Healing Clinic. Hawayo Takata stayed in the clinic for several months, receiving daily Reiki treatments, and as her health returned, she wanted to learn Reiki herself. At first she was not accepted as a student, and she realized that she had to show a deep inner commitment to Reiki. She went to Hayashi and told him about her feelings and her readiness to stay in Japan as long as necessary. Dr. Hayashi agreed that she was ready, and her training began.

Hawayo Takata and her two daughters stayed with the Hayashi family for one year. She gave daily Reiki treatments and continued to study and learn. When her training was finished, she returned to Hawaii with the gift of healing hands.

She became a successful healer in Hawaii. In 1938, Dr. Hayashi and his daughter visited Hawaii and, in February of that year, gave Takata further training and initiated her as a Master of the Usui System of Natural Healing before returning to Japan with his daughter.

In 1941, Hayashi foresaw there would be a war between the United States and Japan, but could not reconcile his work as a Reiki Master with his expected service in the Japanese Marines. At this time, Hawayo Takata had a dream that prompted her to visit Hayashi in Japan. They talked about the war they anticipated, and where she should go to protect herself and the teachings of Reiki.

When everything had been discussed between them and they had agreed on a way to proceed, Hayashi named Hawayo Takata as his successor. He said his goodbyes to everyone and then, dressed in customary Japanese tradition, he sat in the lotus position, closed his eyes, and left his body.

Takata returned to Hawaii as Reiki Master. She became known as a powerful healer and teacher who introduced the gift of Reiki to the Western world. As far as is known, she was the only living Reiki Master until 1976, when she began to train and initiate some of her students to become Reiki Masters. From then until her death in 1980 she initiated twenty-one Reiki Masters, including her grand-daughter Phyllis Lei Furumoto.

Phyllis had received 1st Degree Reiki Initiation as a child. Later, in the 1970s, she received the 2nd Degree initiation. In the spring of 1979, Phyllis was initiated as a Reiki Master and began to travel with her grandmother Takata, receiving intensive lessons and training as her grandmother explained that she was to become her successor as Carrier of the lineage.

Shortly before Takata's death in December 1980, Phyllis received the trust to continue the spiritual Reiki lineage as the Carrier of the lineage.

In the spring of 1982, a group of Reiki Masters gathered in Hawaii with Phyllis Lei Furumoto to honor the memory of Hawayo Takata and they agreed to meet yearly. At the second meeting, "The Reiki Alliance" was founded. The main objective of the conference was to acknowledge Phyllis Lei Furumoto as the successor in direct spiritual descent from Mikao Usui, Chujiro Hayashi, and Hawayo Takata.

The authors were also initiated by Phyllis Lei Furumoto: Brigitte Müller in 1983 in Canada and Horst Günther in July of 1985 in the United States. It means very much to us both to keep to the tradition of Usui's teachings and pass it on.

In the spring of 1988, Phyllis Lei Furumoto gave her blessing and empowerment to those Reiki Masters who felt ready and able to train and initiate new Reiki Masters. Any Masters (Teachers) who take on this enormous responsibility need to have several years of Reiki workshop experience. They must have also the requisite knowledge, skill, and energy to support the Master students they initiate.

In the last few years, Reiki has spread unusually fast around the world. This will contribute to the fulfillment of the world's desire for healing, harmony, love, and brotherhood, and will ultimately bring peace to the whole planet.

3

IN MEMORY OF
MRS. HAWAYO TAKATA

We know that Hawayo Takata played a powerful role in the transmission of Reiki. Because she grew up in Hawaii, Reiki was not lost to the Western Hemisphere as a secret Japanese art, or lost altogether through the Second World War. We remember and honor her with special gratitude.

The following is an excerpt from an interview with Hawayo Takata printed in *The Times* of San Mateo, May 17, 1975:

Reiki? What is Reiki? Mrs. Hawayo (which means Hawaii) Takata, 74, of Hawaii, the Master of Reiki explains: "Reiki means Universal Life Energy." It is not a religion. "It was explained to me this way: 'Here is the great space which surrounds us—the Universe. There is endless and enormous energy in it. It is universal . . . its ultimate source is the Creator. . . . It is a limitless force. It is the source of energy that makes the plants grow, the birds fly.'

Mrs. Takata adds in her words, "It is Nature. It is God, the power He makes available to His children who seek it. In Japanese this is Reiki."

Skeptics may quit now. It is interesting to note, however, that Mrs. Takata points out that the American Medical Association of Hawaii permits Reiki treatments in hospitals, whenever requested by a patient. Also, Mrs. Takata will teach Reiki at the University of Hawaii this winter, for which she has a signed contract. She is living proof that something is very right. At age 74 she plays nine holes of golf daily when at home and participates in 18-hole golf tournaments. She is tiny—and mighty, projecting tranquility, quiet strength and power.

She was not always so. Mrs. Takata recalls when she was 29 her husband died and she was left penniless with two small daughters. "By the time I was 35 I had all kinds of ailments, appendicitis, a benign tumor, gallstones, and to top it, I had asthma, so could not undergo an operation requiring anesthetic. I lost so much weight. Over a period of seven years I was further emotionally devastated; one dear member of my family died each year. I was a church-going woman and had always believed in God. One day I meditated and finally said 'God, I am up against the wall...Help me.' I said to myself, 'If God hears, He will help...'As far as I am concerned, that is what happened. I heard a voice. Today we call that clairaudience. I didn't know anything about that in 1935. I heard a voice speak after I complained so bitterly. I felt all alone in the world, as if I alone had all the suffering, burdens, and poverty. I had said 'Why am I poor? Why do I have such illness and pain? Why do I have all the sorrows?' The voice which replied was loud and clear; it spoke three times. It said 'No—Get rid of all your illness. Just like that you will find health, happiness and security.'

"I couldn't believe my ears until I heard the same message three times. Within 21 days I was on a boat to Tokyo, hoping to find help there. I went to the Maeda Orthopedic Hospital in the district of Akasaka in Tokyo. That is the finest district in the heart of Tokyo near the Royal Palace. The hospital was named after my friend, Dr. T. Maeda, whom I went to see."

Mrs. Takata says that when Dr. Maeda saw her, she was down to 97 pounds. He shook his head and said she would have to build up her strength before any thought of surgery. She and her two small daughters stayed at the hospital. After 21 days in the hospital, Mrs. Takata was ready for surgery and was on the operating table being prepared when suddenly she again heard the commanding voice. This time it said "Do not have the operation. It is not necessary."

Mrs. Takata said she pinched herself to make sure she was both conscious and sane. Three times she heard the admonition and suddenly got off the operating table and stood on the floor causing great consternation among the nurses. Dr. Maeda came in and she told him she was not afraid of dying but wanted to know if there was any other form of treatment. The doctor asked how long she would stay in Japan and when she told him two years, he told the nurse to dress her and called his sister, Mrs. Shimura, and then the hospital dietician.

Mrs. Takata later learned Mrs. Shimura had nearly died of dysentery years before and was in a coma when she was taken to the Reiki Master, Dr. Chijuro Hayashi. She had a miraculous recovery. Now Mrs. Shimura took Mrs. Takata to Dr. Hayashi's offices. "Two of his practitioners worked on me" she recalls. "One treated on the head, sinus, the thyroid, thymus glands; the other on the rest of the body. I can best describe it as it is referred to in the Bible, the 'laying on of hands.' The Maeda Hospital had not yet forwarded my medical history, but they diagnosed my illness perfectly. On my third treatment, my curiosity became boundless. I didn't know what to think. I was obviously improving. I was still staying at the Maeda Hospital where they checked and confirmed my progress.

"I am a very curious woman. I said to myself, 'I am going to investigate how they are doing this. What makes me feel first the warmth then actual heat emanating from these hands? I looked under the table, at the ceiling, everywhere. I could find no cords or instruments. Then I thought, 'Aha, they have a battery hidden in their sleeves.' Dr. Hayashi's assistants wore the Japanese kimono with long sleeves which hold pockets. They worked so silently. There was no talking. My moment came. When I was being treated, I suddenly grabbed the practitioner by the pocket. He was startled, but thinking I needed some tissue, he thoughtfully handed me some. I said, 'No, I want to see the machine in your pocket.' He burst into loud laughter. Dr. Hayashi came in to see what the commotion was all about. "He smiled and shook his head Mrs. Takata recalls. He proceeded to give her the explanation of a Universal Life Force. He said, "Whenever you feel the contact, all I know is that I have reached this great Universal Life Force and it comes through me to you—these are the electrodes," and he held up his hands. "That force begins to revitalize and restore the balance of your entire system."

In time Mrs. Takata became convinced she too, should learn more and become a student of Dr. Hayashi. She adds, "I passed my examinations perfectly."

"I speak with confidence about this," Mrs. Takata notes, "but please understand I do not speak as 'I'—I speak because it is God's power. He is the One who makes it available to us. "Mrs. Takata is the only teacher of the Usui system of Reiki in the world today and she is recognized as its Master. (1975)

HAWAYO TAKATA'S RECIPES

Mrs. Takata had her own health recipes. The following are two of her recommendations:

—m—

GARDEN SALAD

1 small cabbage finely cut

2–3 medium-size red beets, grated raw

4 celery sticks, finely cut

1 small head of cauliflower, finely cut

1 apple (can be added for a special taste variation)

This makes a very large serving. It is recommended to reduce the size of the ingredients to make a fresh salad every day.

TAKATA'S REJUVENATING DRINK

1 grapefruit

3 small red beets, peeled

2 handfuls of cut cabbage

$1^1/_2$ cups of water

4 tablespoons peeled almonds

4 tablespoons sunflower seeds

Mix in blender until completely liquid, and then add 6 tablespoons Lecithin powder and 2 tablespoons brewers yeast. Now take half of this mixture and add a half gallon of spring water. Drink several glasses daily.

4

How to Become
a Reiki Channel

Previous experience is not necessary to become a Reiki practitioner, but the healing power of Reiki can, in general, only be *transmitted* through a Reiki Master/Teacher. A person should have an open heart, the desire to receive the Reiki transmission and carry the intention to use it. If a student wants to heal themselves and their family, other people, animals, or plants, then the channel will open for the healing energy during the Reiki instruction.

Preparation and Initiation for the 1st Degree

The 1st Degree is given over a weekend, or on four consecutive days or evenings, in sessions lasting three to four hours each. Sometimes it will also be given in a holiday workshop. During the workshop, the Reiki Master/Teacher undertakes four initiations or "power transmissions." These will prepare the students and open their inner healing channels. Each initiation is a blessing and healing. What happens is a kind of a cleansing on all levels, affecting the body, mind, and soul, and raising the vibrational frequency of all participants. Blocks and toxins are released, and healing is encouraged. The transmission of energy may also cause self-healing reactions which will mostly cease after the workshop.

You will receive the basic training and hand positions to give yourself Reiki. Often participants feel the flow of Reiki after the first initiation and learn to exchange the universal life energy with other members of the workshop. Reiki flows depending on the need of the receiver, who only takes as much as needed. You feel clearly that you only act as a channel and that none of your own energy is taken. On the contrary, you are being charged simultaneously and self-healing is taking place. The flow of this loving, healing, gentle, and powerful energy is an uplifting experience.

Reiki will change your life, and accelerate your mental and physical healing as well as your spiritual growth, so you will clearly feel the connection with your inner self and you will touch yourself with love. Because of this, you will be in harmony and peace with yourself and the world. Reiki also helps you have the courage to change those things in your life that you want to change. By the end of the workshop you have received the gift of healing hands. Every person heals themselves. Now you have the tools to do so. Take responsibility for yourself, change your thoughts and behavior according to the "Spiritual Rules of Life," and you will become a new human being with much more joy in life.

Preparation and Initiation for the 2nd Degree.

Traditionally, the Usui System of Reiki is taught in two degrees. When you have completed the 1st Degree and have used Reiki actively in your life, then you can deepen your connection with Reiki and your own spiritual growth through the initiation into the 2nd Degree. At least three months should pass between the initiations of the 1st and the 2nd Degree. Only in exceptional cases can you receive the 2nd Degree earlier. Within yourself, you should feel when the time is right to receive the 2nd Degree, as there will be much movement on many levels. Be ready for further change in your life.

The 2nd Degree is called *Oku Den*, or "deep knowledge," and is a psychic opening. It will especially act on subtle people. Your intuition and ability to heal will expand. With your initiation, you receive the secret holy symbols and the specific mantras. These are solely for the use of people initiated into the 2nd Degree. Their use carries a large responsibility.

Through the initiation into the 2nd Degree, the healing powers are increased and intensified, and you learn to use the symbols to give mental healing and to heal over a distance independent of space and time. Mental healing means you now possess the ability to connect yourself with the sub- and higher consciousness, or your Higher Self, and to initiate healing through the spirit, for example in cases of depression, sleeplessness, nervous breakdowns, and addictions. You can also use mental healing on yourself to change rigid patterns of behavior into new, constructive ones.

You become aware that you carry the responsibility for your life and that you are the master of your life and your circumstances. Since everyone is on the way to mastering themselves, whether it is conscious or not, and everyone needs to learn how to use these energies wisely. Everything you send out comes back to you (the Law of the Circle). If you send out much joy and love, it will return many times over. Thus it is very important that you take responsibility for the enhanced energy you possess after the 2nd Degree initiation.

5

Becoming a Reiki Master/Teacher

In the spring of 1988, Phyllis Lei Furumoto gave her blessing and authorization for the initiation of Masters to all those Reiki Masters who felt willing and able to train and initiate others.

The call to become a Reiki Master/Teacher is intuitively recognized by those people who have been initiated in the 1st and 2nd Degree and who have practiced for some time. The initiation brings along with it further personal growth and change on all levels.

We, the authors received the blessing and authorization to carry out this training through the initiation and relationship established with Phyllis Lei Furumoto. In great gratitude, we now have brought several Reiki Masters/Teachers onto this path. We are completely aware of the unending responsibility the Master accepts in initiating a student to the level of a Master/Teacher.

The program of the training is individually tailored to the individual needs of the person who is ready for this further step.

Suggestions for Reiki Practitioners

R eiki flows and works only through the hands of a practitioner who has received the four initiations of the 1st Degree, or after that, the initiations into the 2nd Degree through an authorized Reiki Master/ Teacher. Only with these initiations are students empowered to give Reiki to themselves or others. In case you have not received a Reiki initiation, we hope the following descriptions and pictures will be informative and inspiring.

Due to the protection of the initiations, the Reiki practitioner only acts as a channel and simply transmits the universal life energy, so that no personal energy is taken from him. He himself will even be enriched with energy.

For all those who have taken part in a Reiki workshop and are Reiki channels, the following guide to Reiki treatment will serve to deepen their knowledge. It is not important to follow the exact order of the hand positions, but rather let yourselves be guided by Reiki, which works by intuition. In our many years of experience in treatment and workshops, the following descriptions have proven to be highly successful, and in general we can say, "Let Reiki guide your hands to the right position."

SELF–HEALING WITH REIKI

After you have received the Reiki initiation of the 1st Degree, you should give Reiki to yourself every day to strengthen your health and to charge your *life battery* with energy. This will maintain your physical and mental health, support your spiritual growth, and expand your awareness. You become whole, giving yourself love and handling your stress and daily commitments better. In her workshops, Hawayo Takata always recommended beginning with yourself.

"You are number one," she said, "and if you still have time afterwards you can give Reiki to your family and friends." You should first love and heal yourself because you are only capable of giving to others what you would give to yourself. This is the deeper meaning of saying, "love your neighbor as you love yourself."

The more intensively you use Reiki, the stronger the energy grows within you. Simply get used to putting your hands onto your body whenever they are free, for example:

- In the morning after waking up, to activate and balance your chakras (this is especially intensive with the use of the 2nd Degree symbols).

- During the day when making phone calls, in the subway, during rush hour, while watching TV, in the theater, during waiting periods, and so forth.

- At night in bed, to help fall asleep or to sleep through the night.

Reiki can be very helpful in overcoming alcohol or drug addiction, since it reaches deeper levels of awareness. Reiki of the 2nd Degree, especially, can reach the subconscious mind and transmit the universal life energy onto another level. It is also recommended that positive affirmations be included in the mental treatment of the 2nd Degree.

Give yourself a full Reiki treatment whenever possible. You will become healed and complete in body, mind, and spirit.

If a time comes when you don't want to give Reiki to yourself or others, it might be because you have a resistance to your growth and change. In this case, it would be good to continue with Reiki as it will release this resistance. Reiki will give you the courage to shape your life the way you like it. All you need to do is give yourself Reiki every day. Reiki is the teacher.

Head Position Self-Healing: H

H 1—Eyes/Sinuses

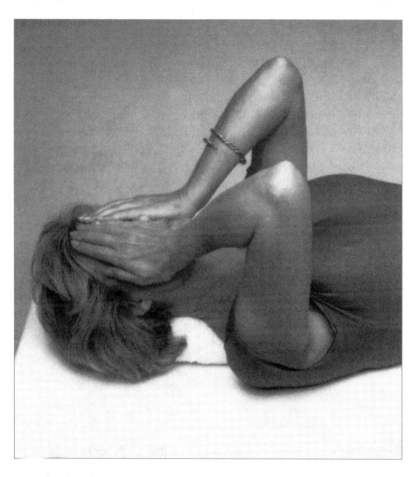

Over forehead, eyes and cheeks. Eye problems, gray and green cataract sinuses • head cold • allergies • asthma • cerebral nerves • pituitary gland • pineal gland.

Balances the pituitary and pineal glands. The pineal gland is the central point of hormonal regulation. Very relaxing in stress situations. The 6th chakra (third eye) relates to the 1st chakra.

H 2A—To the Sides of the Temples

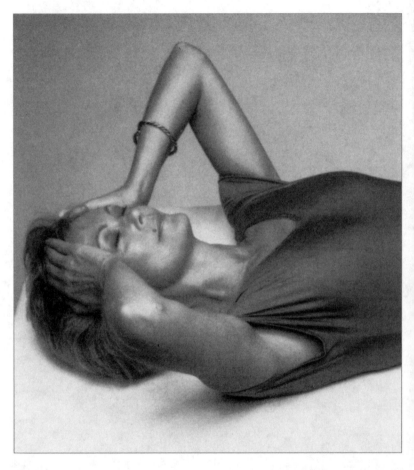

To the sides of the temples, optic nerves. Balances the right brain (intuition, wisdom) and the left brain (rational understanding). Very relaxing in stress situations.

H 2B—Ears

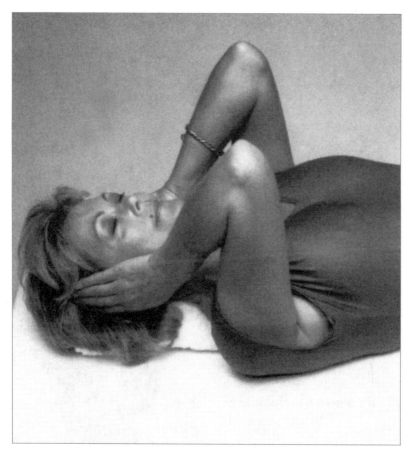

Over the ears. Many organs can be treated around the ears (acupuncture points: heart, intestines, kidneys, lungs, stomach, liver, or gallbladder.). Used for colds and flu, hearing problems, buzzing noises in the ear, loss of balance.

H 3—Back of the Head

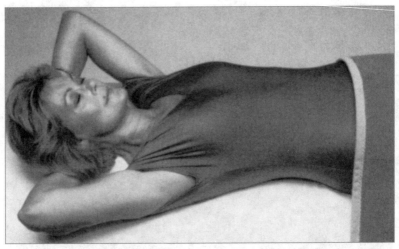

Back of the head, onto medulla oblongata. Eyes • vision • headaches, • nosebleeds • hay fever, sinuses • stroke • digestion • fear • shock, • worries. Will calm and clear thoughts. Medulla oblongata is connected to the third eye

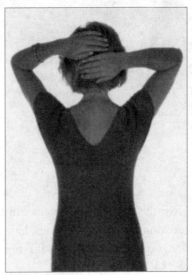

H 4—*Top of the Head*

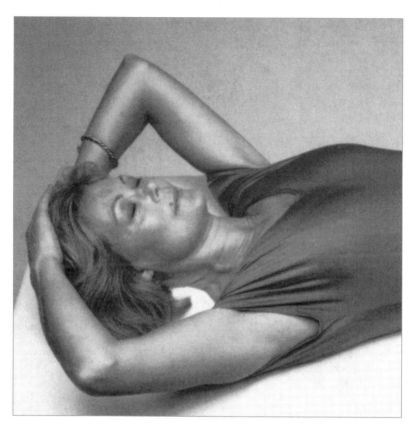

Across the head. Headaches • eye pains • abdominal cramps • flatulence and digestion problems • bladder • multiple sclerosis • stress and emotions. • 7th chakra.

H 5—Thyroid Gland • Thymus Gland

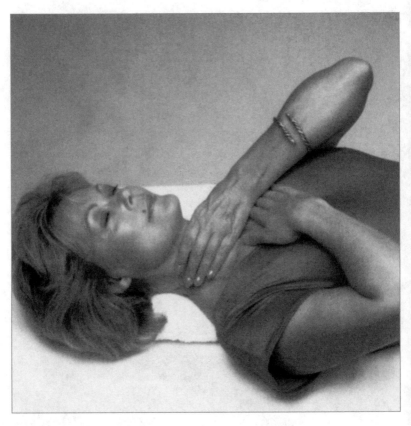

On the sides and the front of the throat. Thyroid gland • important for metabolism • over or underweight • palpitation • angina • flu • high or low blood pressure • anger • frustration • communication • self–expression. 5th chakra, related to the 2nd chakra.

Special Position—Eyes and Teeth

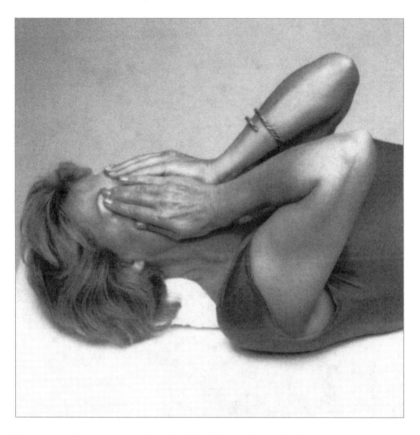

Eyes • teeth • sinuses. For head colds and toothaches.

Special Position—Eyes

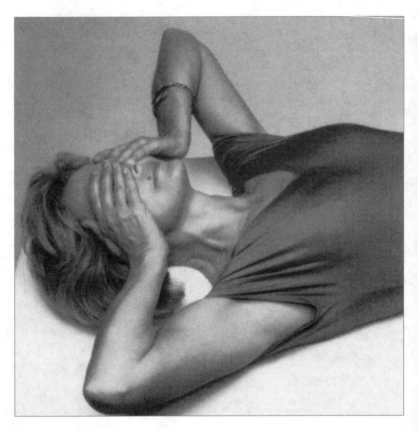

Eyes • sinuses.

Special Position—To Focus

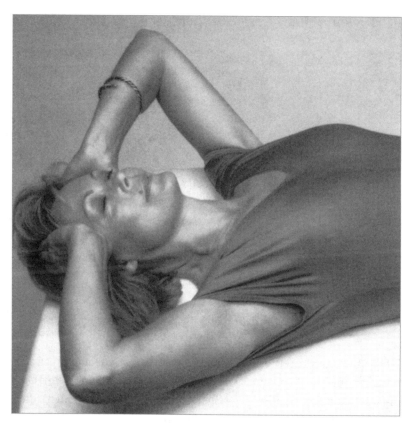

To balance the left and right brain, in cases of stress, headaches.

Basic Position Self–Healing (Front): BP

BP 1—Right Side, Liver/Gall (with G 2 left side)

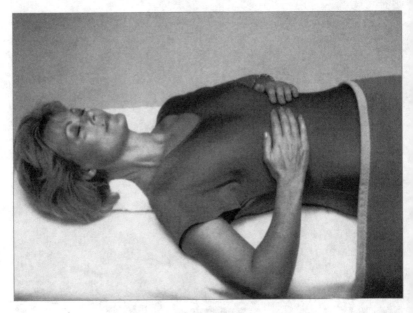

Under the chest. Liver • gallbladder • part of the stomach • pancreas • spleen anemia • leukemia • immune system • infections • AIDS • cancer • jaundice • gallstones • hypoglycemia • diabetes • detoxification • sorrow • anger • depression • suppressed chronic complaints • loss of balance

BP 2—Left Side, Pancreas (with G 1 right side)

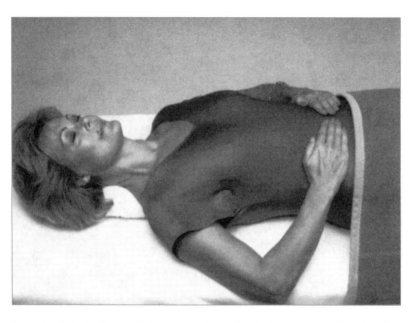

At waist height. Part of the stomach • tail of the pancreas (production of insulin and enzymes) • large intestine • small intestine • anemia • leukemia • immune system • diabetes • flu • infections • AIDS • cancer

BP 3—Solar Plexus

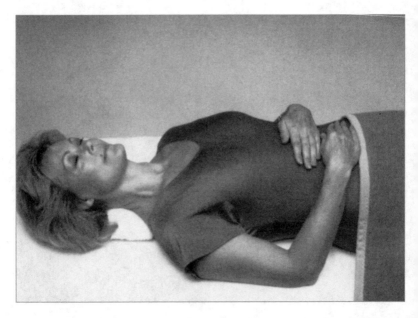

Upper hand on the stomach, lower hand on the navel. Solar plexus
• stomach intestines • heart • digestion • lymph • shock • emotions •
depression

The Hara is approximately 1 inch under the navel, energy center. 2nd
and 3rd chakra.

BP 4—V Position Abdomen

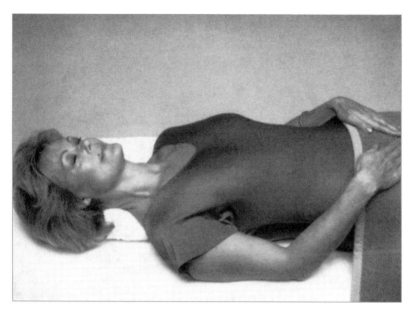

On the abdomen, V position. Organs of the abdomen • intestines • ovaries • bladder • urethra • cardiovascular • digestion • appendix (right) • breast tumors • cramps • menopause complication • backaches • tumors in the ovaries/uterus/bladder. 1st and 2nd chakra

BP 5—Heart/Thymus

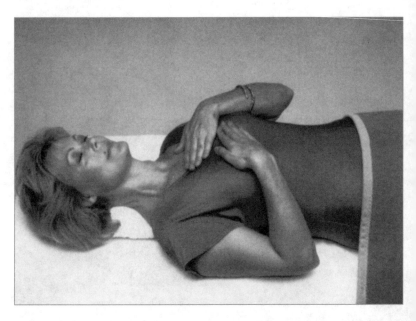

In the Heart Position. Heart • thymus gland • lung • heart ailments •
bronchitis • immune system • lymph • deafness • emotions • depression. 4th chakra

Special Positions Self–Healing

Special Position—Thighs (inner side)

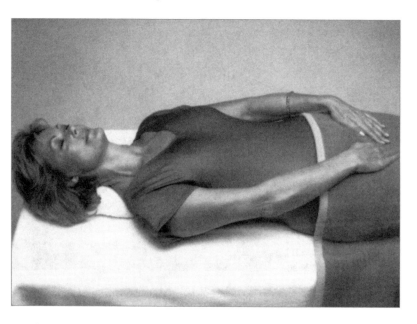

On the inner side of the thigh. Blood circulation.

Special Position—Greater Trochanter—Legs/Gallbladder

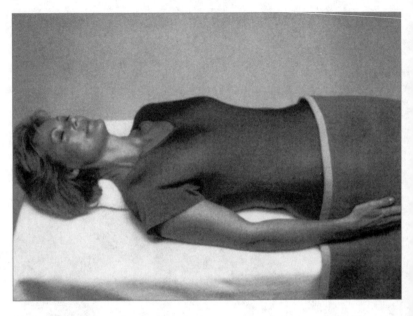

Greater trochanter. Varicose veins • leg pain • gall point

Special Position—Breasts

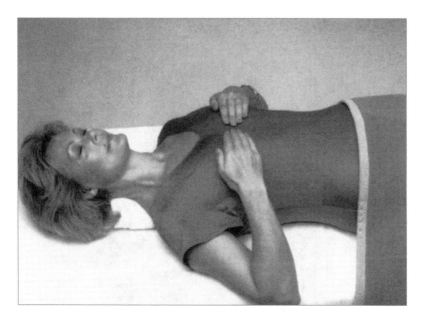

On both breasts. (If not appropriate, give Reiki a few inches away).

Back Position Self–Healing: B

B 1—Shoulders/Neck

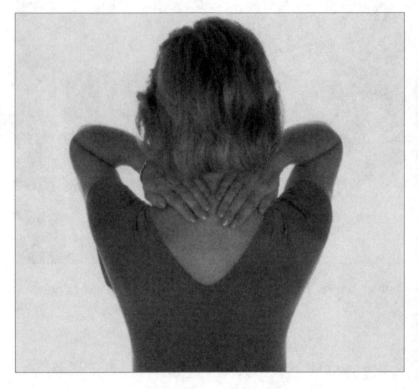

On the shoulders. Left and right on the shoulders • For stress and tightness

B 1A—7th Vertebra (Medulla Oblongata)

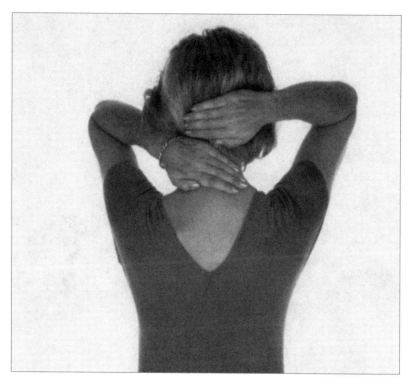

In the neck/7th vertebra (medulla oblongata). For pain in the bones, heart • vertebrae • nerves • shock on the spine • neck problems

B 3—Kidneys/Adrenal Glands

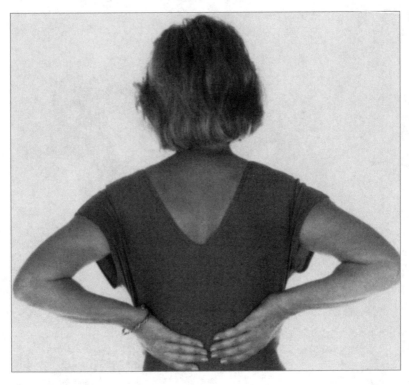

Nerves • heart • lung • adrenal glands • backaches • shock • allergies • hay fever • stress • detoxification • and as performed on the front of the body

B 4—Waist

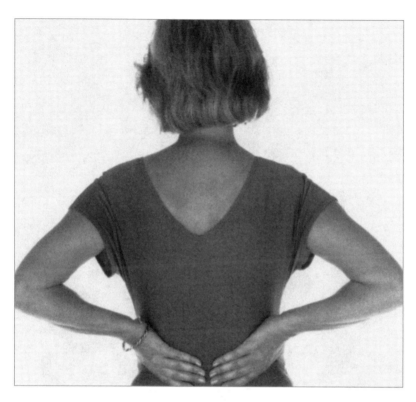

Around the waist. Nerves•lung • kidneys • backaches • shock • allergies • hay fever • stress • detoxification • and as performed on the
front of the body

B 5—Hip

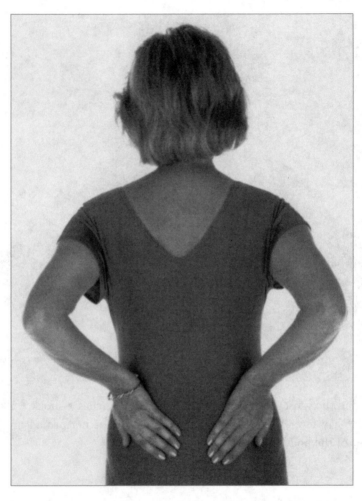

On the hips. Sciatica • lymph • nerves • backaches • hip •
and as performed on the front of the body

B 6—Buttocks

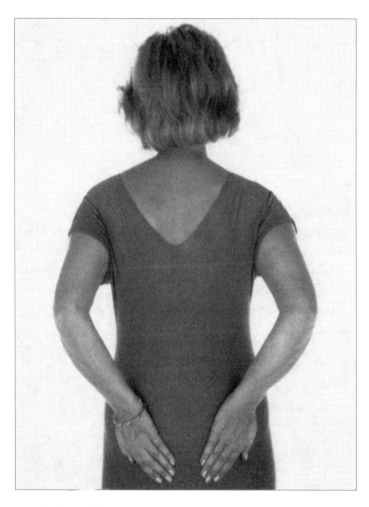

On the buttocks. Sciatica • lymph • nerves • backaches • hips
• and as performed on the front of the body

8

ANATOMIC
ILLUSTRATIONS

In general, it is not necessary to know a great deal about human anatomy or the anatomy of animals in order to give a Reiki treatment. However, it can be very helpful, especially when wanting to treat certain organs more specifically. Following are simple anatomic illustrations of the bodies of humans, dogs, cats, and horses. For further studies we recommend an anatomic atlas.

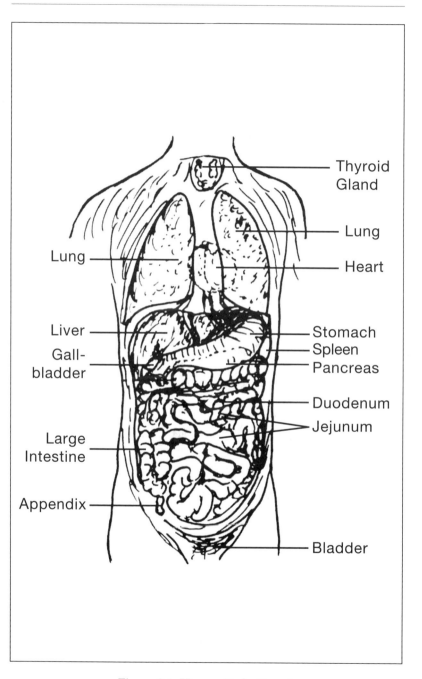

Figure 8.1. Human Body (Front)

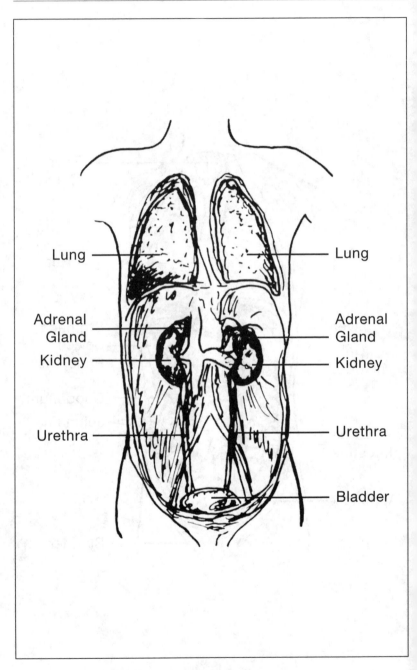

Figure 8.2. The Human Body (Back)

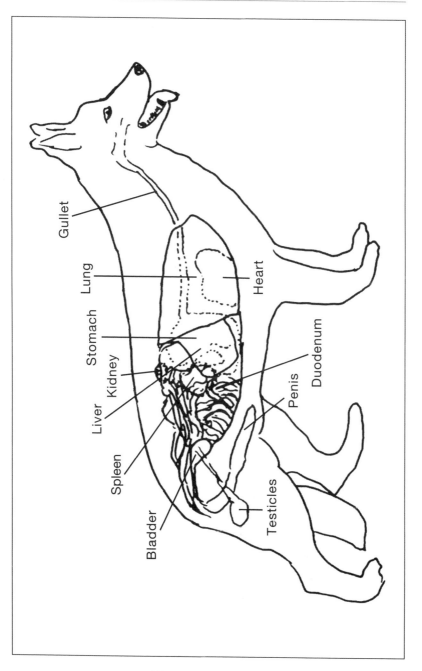

Figure 8.3. The Dog

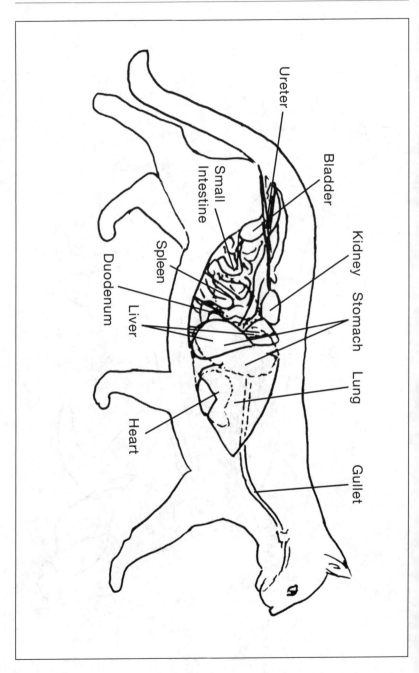

Figure 8.4. The Cat

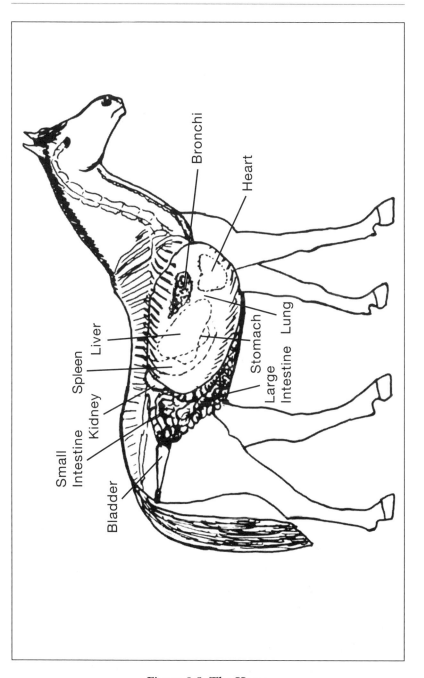

Figure 8.5. The Horse

9

RECOMMENDATIONS FOR REIKI TREATMENT

General Recommendations

A complete Reiki treatment is always given except in emergencies and accidents, or when a quick treatment is needed. This is because not only the symptoms, but also the *cause* of an ailment are in need of a treatment in order to bring about a complete healing process. The person giving Reiki is only a channel and thus has no influence on the result of the treatment. This responsibility for healing lies solely within the receiving person, and on a deep level which cannot be consciously controlled. When the receiver is ready and open for the healing process, then his or her self-healing powers are activated through Reiki. The person giving Reiki should be aware that it is not a personal achievement when healing occurs, but is the result of a divine force. Hence, it is crucial to understand that you *do everything right* when giving a Reiki treatment, you cannot do anything wrong. It's not necessary to analyze this, either, since a reaction in the hands will indicate when the cause of the problem has been found—for example, it could be perceived as a hot or cold feeling. The hands should stay on these places until the energy flow is normalized.

The faith of the Reiki practitioner strengthens the healing power, thus each channel will be tested as to the degree of belief. However, doubts and/or unwillingness can reduce the effectiveness of the practitioner's ability to administer Reiki. Since Reiki becomes stronger as it is used, it is important to use Reiki often; it's also important because, like an unused muscle, it will atrophy if not used. However, Reiki should only be used to help and heal. If it is used with the wrong intention, it will not work.

At the start of a series of Reiki treatments, the practitioner should, if possible, give four treatments on four consecutive days. These four days give the body the opportunity to free itself from its toxins. During this time it is possible to have strong self-healing reactions, so that chronic ailments often appear temporarily. It can also trigger emotional reactions, which are to be judged positively. These kinds of reactions to Reiki healing usually recede within twelve to twenty-four hours. After the initial four days, further treatments can be given once or twice a week, or even daily over a period of several weeks, to allow the person's self-healing powers to flow.

In general, a Reiki treatment takes about one to one and a half hours, so the practitioner remains in each position for about three to five minutes depending on the energy flow. Specific problems or pain areas can be treated for an extra ten to twenty minutes or even longer. In urgent cases, a treatment can last several hours or can be repeated several times a day.

There are exceptions to the duration of a treatment. For example, it is best to give Reiki to older or very sensitive people for only about thirty minutes initially, increasing the time as they get used to it. Twenty to thirty minutes is also enough with small children.

Reiki flows through clothing, plaster, belts, and bandages, and similar, so it is not necessary to undress before a treatment. You should be in a quiet space of mind and create a peaceful atmosphere during the treatment, and conversations should usually be avoided, except when psychotherapeutic sessions are combined with Reiki. Calming, meditative music can be very supportive during treatment.

Reiki does not replace a medical doctor's care or medication. However, it supports any kind of therapy and the natural healing processes, as it activates self-healing powers. It is especially helpful before and after surgery; it strengthens, harmonizes, and calms the patient, accelerating recovery and helping the wound to heal faster and better. By giving yourself Reiki before and after surgery with local anesthesia, or at the dentist, you can achieve a soothing effect. You should not give yourself Reiki *directly* after the anesthesia or during the procedure, however, as our experience shows this can reduce, delay, or prematurely cancel the anesthesia.

Chronic ailments take much longer to improve and require repeated treatments of several hours duration over a longer period of time. In cases of immediate, severe sickness (for example AIDS or cancer), Reiki should be given daily for several hours. This means ideally that members of the family should be initiated into Reiki to perhaps give treatments in twenty-four-hour shifts (see also description in Chapter 3). In contrast to chronic ailments, you can usually see a positive change in accident victims very quickly.

If circumstances do not allow multiple Reiki treatments, then the rule becomes "a little Reiki is always better than none." At the end of a Reiki treatment, please remember that you only function as a channel, no matter what happened during the treatment. Be thankful that the healing power was able to flow through you—it is an appropriate time for a prayer of gratitude for grace received.

Practical Details

- Take off watches and rings.

- Wash your hands with soap before and after the treatment.

- Loosen tight belts, waistbands, and neckties (on the Reiki receiver as well).

- The receiver should take his/her shoes off and lie relaxed without crossing the legs.

- Quiet, meditative music, which has healing qualities, helps relax the receiver.

- Use a blanket and put a fresh tissue over the eyes.

- Begin by making the connection between you and the universal life energy, so you can function as a healing channel.

- Stroke the aura three times to smooth it (in a circle from the head to the feet and back). This is relaxing. However, be careful to move your arm close to your body when you go from the feet back to the head, otherwise you will stroke against the aura.

- Sit in a comfortable, relaxed position.

- Apply your hands without pressure, slightly arched, matching the shape of the body, so that you make good contact.

- It is very helpful for the receiver if she/he feels or breathes into the parts that you touch.

- Maintain continuous contact between the hands and the body after the treatment has begun, even when changing into the next position. Do not remove your hands from the person without first telling them.

- Keep your fingers close together.

- If your hands do not always feel *hot*, it does not mean that Reiki is not flowing. The energy flow depends on the needs of the receiver who absorbs as much energy as needed. This can vary from session to session.

- Sometimes the receiver falls asleep during the treatment. This is actually an advantage, because the energy can flow freely without being consciously influenced by the mind.

- If organs or limbs are missing, give Reiki in these areas as if they were there. For example, treat an artificial limb and the remaining stump.

- If there is a cast, put your hands on it. Reiki flows through the cast.

- In case of burns, hold your hands over the injured area at some distance, letting your receiver know you are lifting your hands off the body for that part of the treatment.

- It is a good idea to let the receiver know that conditions can sometimes worsen after the first Reiki treatment due to possible self-healing reactions and emotions. However, these feelings will generally pass within twelve to twenty-four hours.

- Before you reach the end of a session, ask the receiver if there is any place that still wants to be treated.

- To finish a session, put your hands in the arch of the knees and on the feet (fingertips touching the tips of the toes) to become grounded.

- Apply a hand on the person's back and stroke the aura to smooth it three times. You can also draw a line of energy from the posterior to the head. Afterwards, express your gratefulness to the Universal Source.

- Think of Reiki in emergencies and accidents. Your hands are always ready to heal.

The key word for Reiki is simplicity. Let Reiki flow from your inner self. Be in your heart. Reiki will intuitively lead you to the places that need energy. Don't necessarily feel bound to the hand positions you've been taught. Reiki will develop your inner knowledge. Follow the lead of your hands. Reiki will lead you.

Reiki energy is within you,
The Divine is the origin and the source.
You are connected to the source.
Reiki is unconditional love.

10

SPECIAL PERCEPTIONS AND REACTIONS DURING REIKI TREATMENTS

Reiki energy refines and increases perceptions and sensibilities. The person giving the Reiki treatment may have special sensations during a treatment, and some reactions about the client may be transmitted to them, intuitively leading them to the places that require special attention. This makes it possible to not only treat the visible symptoms, but to reach the actual origin of an ailment.

Reactions can occur in both the person giving Reiki and the receiver. The person acting as the Reiki channel is charged with this energy during the treatment and is flooded with healing energy, which allows her or him to perceive a number of sensations: strong warmth or heat in the hands, tingles, vibrations, shaking (at times like electric waves), heat in the entire body, as well as sweat in certain places that become very hot and thus draw in a lot of energy. The energy runs in waves and little by little in cycles. Each cycle can last several minutes, during which the hands stay on that particular spot until the *drawing in* of energy decreases. If it feels as though the hands are glued to the spot, they should definitely stay there longer, between ten and twenty minutes. We know from our own experiences and those of others who, similar to an electrical transformer, alter energy, that we get reactions, such as yawning, coughing, belching, hiccups, strong vibrating, shaking hands, and thirst, when reaching interrupted or blocked areas. We recommend that people who have these or similar reactions while giving Reiki try to not suppress these sensations, but allow them to occur.

If the Reiki receiver starts to cry or laugh during the treatment, it is important to stay with the area that released this emotion until calming sets in. The same is true for heat sensations. In these cases as well, the corresponding positions are treated until they are normalized. In cases of cold sensations, it may be necessary to give Reiki longer and more often, as there could be a chronic problem in these areas.

In the Reiki receiver, it is possible to experience such sensations and reactions as pressure in the head, stings, which suddenly run through the body (for example, a twitch in the leg), feelings of heat or cold, which can be felt differently by the giver and the receiver, emotions, such as laughing or crying, and sightings of light, colors, pictures, and visions.

After the treatment, there may be self-healing reactions of the receiver, such as slight shivers, which will change into a nice feeling of warmth after about ten minutes, an urgent need to use the bathroom, hunger or thirst, chronic ailments, which may become apparent, headaches, pressure in the head, emotions (usually after the 3rd treatment), a change in the condition of the stool and urine (drinking a lot of water helps with detoxification), intensifying pain, for example with broken bones. In a natural healing process, it is common for symptoms to increase first—sometimes it is necessary for the problems to peak before they can leave the body completely—but these self–healing reactions usually pass within twelve to twenty-four hours.

After several Reiki sessions—the number is individually different—the receiver feels *born again*, charged and full of energy, free of pain, relaxed and in harmony, strengthened, balanced, and full of joy and fresh courage to change things in their life.

11

REIKI TREATMENT ILLUSTRATIONS

Reiki Treatment

Stroking the Aura to Smooth It

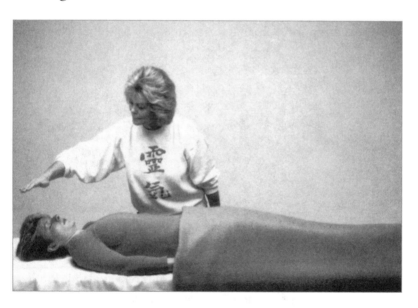

In the beginning of the treatment, you can smooth the aura (the energy field surrounding the body) with oval-shaped strokes as you move from the head to the feet. This is very relaxing. Please be sure that your hands stay close to your body as you move them from the feet up to the head.

Head Position: H

H1—Eyes/Sinuses

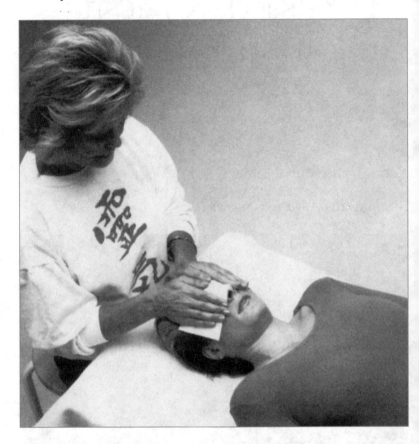

Over the forehead, eyes and cheeks. Eye problems • cataracts • glaucoma • sinuses • colds • allergies • nerves in the brain • pituitary gland • pineal gland. Balances pituitary and pineal gland. Pituitary gland is the center of hormonal regulation. Relaxing in cases of stress and tightness. 6th chakra (third eye), is connected to the 1st chakra.

H 2A—To the Sides of the Temples

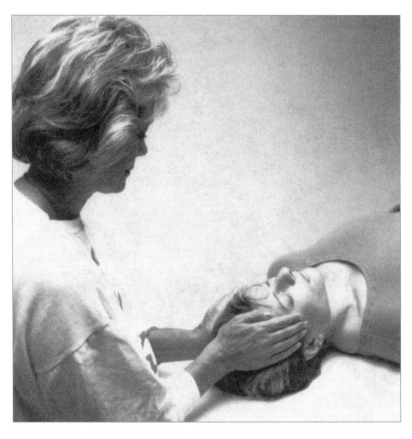

To the sides of the temples. Optic nerves. Balances the right (intuition, wisdom) and the left (rational understanding) sides of the
brain. Very relaxing in cases of stress.

H 2B—Ears

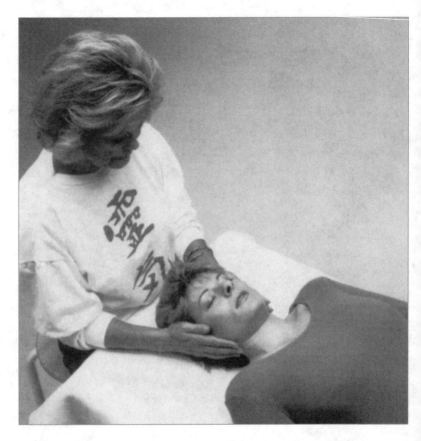

Over the ears. Treatment on the ears covers many organs (acupuncture points include heart, intestines, kidneys, lungs, stomach, liver, gallbladder, and others). In cases of colds and flu, lack of hearing, tinnitus, problems with physical stability.

H 3—Back of the Head

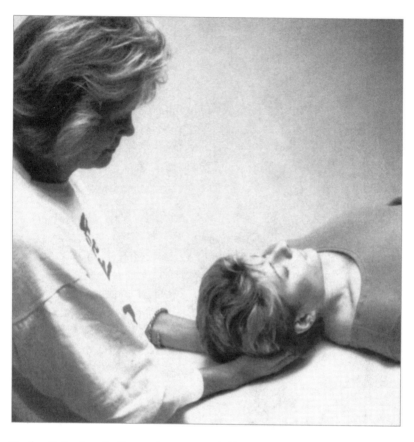

Back of the head, fingertips on medulla oblongata. Eyes • vision • headaches • nose bleeds • hay fever • sinuses • stroke • digestive problems • fear • shock • worries. Calms and clears thoughts. Medulla oblongata is connected to the third eye.

H 4—On the Top of the Head

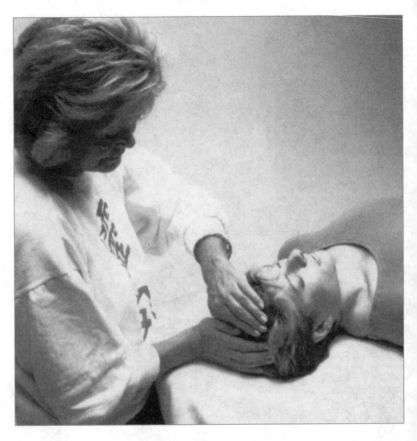

Across the top of the head. Headaches • eye pains • cramps in the abdomen • gas and digestive problems • bladder • multiple sclerosis • stress and emotions. 7th chakra.

H 5—Thyroid Gland/Thymus Gland

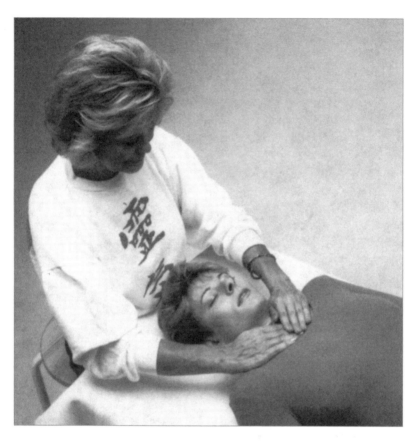

On the sides and front of the throat. Thyroid gland • important for metabolism • over- or underweight • heart pounding and fluttering • sore throat • flu • high or low blood pressure • anger • frustration • communication • self-expression. 5th chakra, connected to the 2nd chakra.

Special Position—Eyes

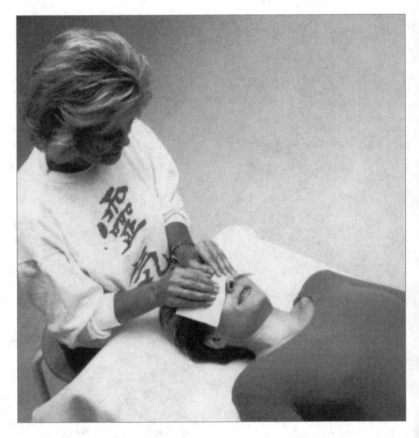

On the eyes. Putting the fingertips very softly on the eyes.

Special Position—Eyes

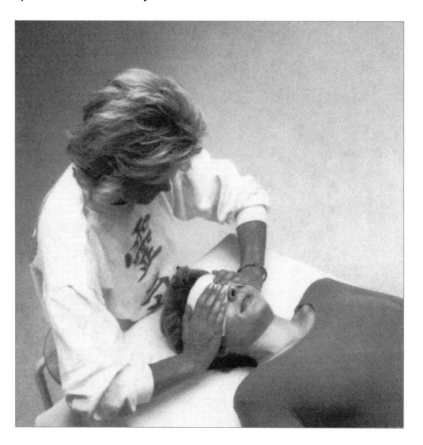

On the eyes. Eye nerves • sinuses

Special Position—To Center

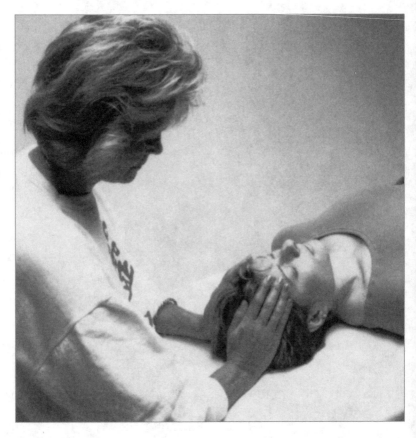

Sylvan fissure/capillary system. In cases of stress • tightness and headaches • to center • problems with balance

Special Position—Motor Nerves

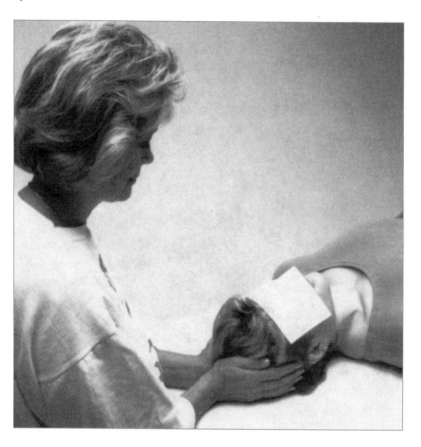

Motor nerves

Special Position—Collarbone

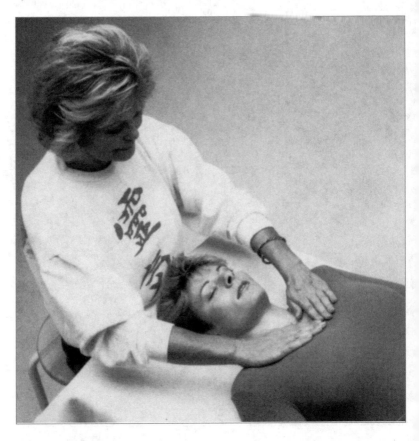

On the collarbone. Bronchial tubes • stress • emotions • asthma • fear • coughing

Special Position—Shoulders

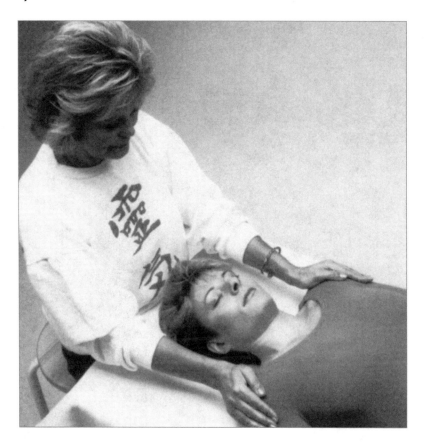

On the shoulders. Pains in the arms • cold hands • disrupted blood flow in the arms

Basic Position (front): BP

BP 1—Right, Liver/Gallbladder

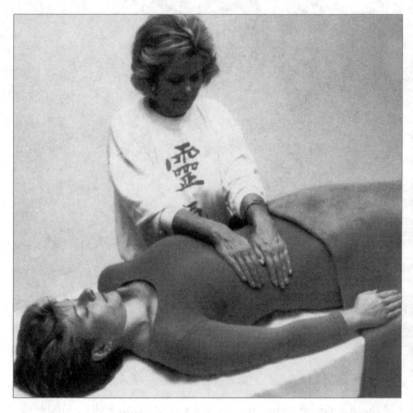

On the right, under the chest/waist. Liver • gallbladder • part of the stomach • pancreas • duodenum • large intestine • jaundice • gallstones • hypoglycemia • diabetes • detoxification • sadness • anger • depression • suppressed chronic illnesses • problems with physical stability

BP 2—Left, Pancreas

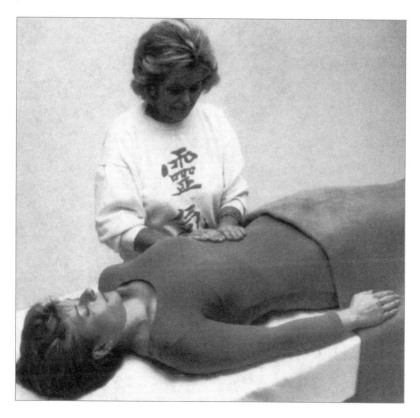

On the left, under the chest/waist. Parts of the stomach • tail of the pancreas (production of insulin and enzymes) • spleen • large intestine • small intestine • anemia • leukemia • immune system • diabetes • flu infection • AIDS • cancer

BP 3—Solar Plexus

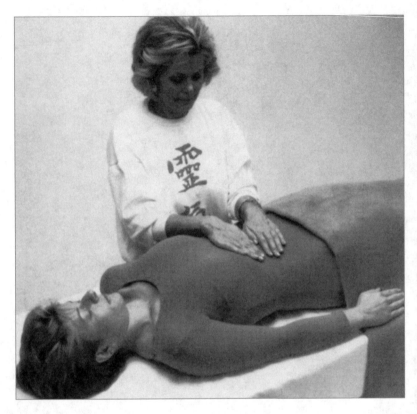

Lower hand on the navel, upper hand on the stomach. Solar plexus • stomach • intestines • heart • digestion • lymph • shock • emotions • depression • Hara, approximately 1 inch under the navel. 3rd chakra.

BP 4—V Position, Abdomen

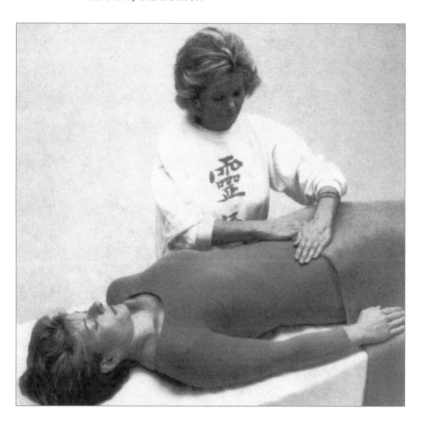

On the abdomen, V Position. Organs in the abdomen • intestines • ovaries • bladder • urethra • blood circulation • digestion • appendix on the right • breast tumors • cramps • menopausal complications • backaches • tumors in the ovaries/uterus/bladder. 1st and 2nd chakra.

BP 5—Heart/Thymus

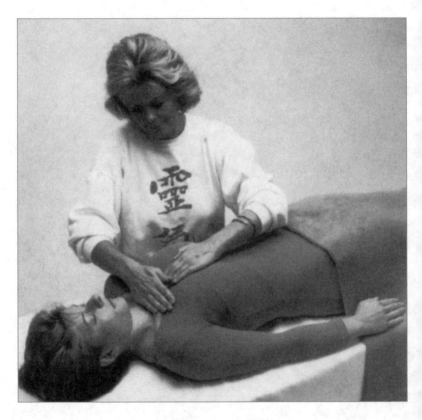

Heart, T Position. Heart • thymus gland • lungs • heart problems • bronchitis • immune system • lymph • deafness • emotions. 4th chakra.

Special Positions

Special Position—Greater Trochanter • Legs/Gallbladder

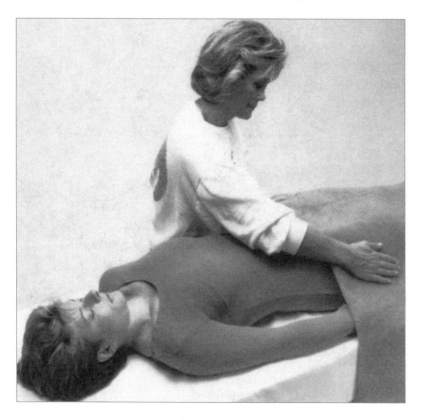

Greater Trochanter. Varicose veins • leg pains • gallbladder point.

Special Position—Breasts

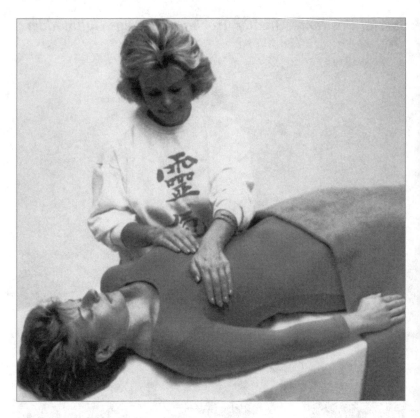

On both breasts. Harmonization of the masculine and feminine sides.

Back Position: B

For B 1–B 6: Both hands together or next to each other, beginning at the shoulders, down to the edge of the buttocks.

B 1—Shoulders

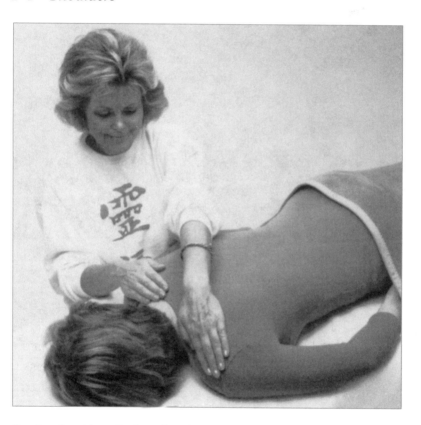

On the shoulders. Left and right on the shoulders • in cases of stress and tightness.

B 1A—7th Vertebra/Medulla Oblongata

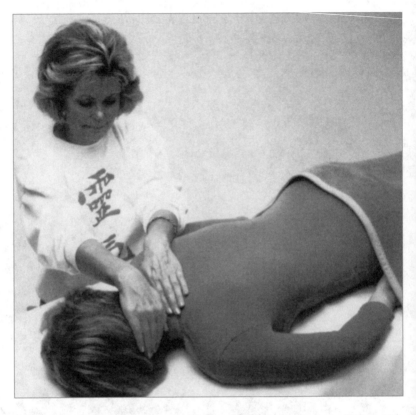

On the neck/7th Vertebra (medulla oblongata). For pain in bones •
heart • vertebrae • nerves • shock on the spine • neck problems

B 2—Lung

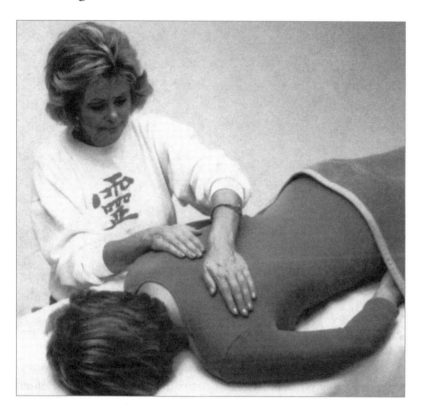

Over the lung. Coughing • bronchitis • stress • neck problems • back and shoulder complications • and as on the front of the body

B 3 and B 4—Kidneys (Adrenal Glands)

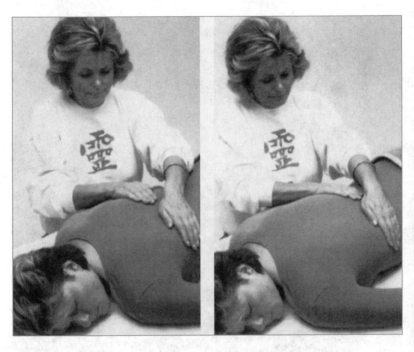

Nerves • heart • lung • adrenal glands • kidneys • backaches • shock • allergies • hay fever • stress • detoxification • in cases of emergencies and accidents • and as on the front of the body

B 5 and B 6—Hip/Buttocks

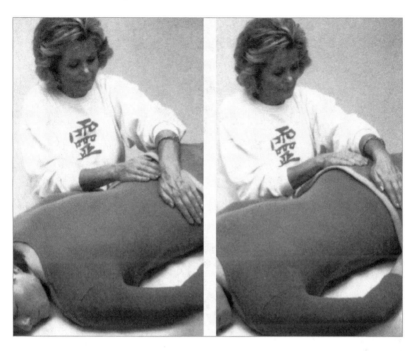

Sciatica • lymph • nerves • backaches • hip • and as the on the front of the body

B 7—T Position

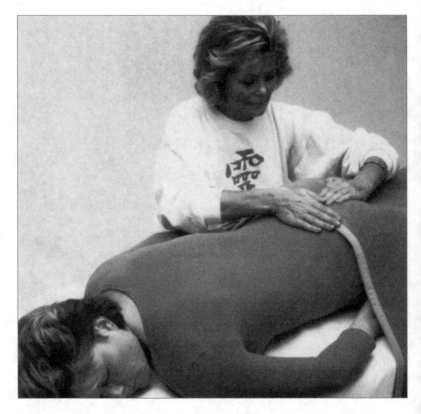

The energy center on the coccyx, 1st chakra. Sciatica • nerves • prostate • vaginal complications • bladder • hemorrhoids • and as on the front of the body

B 8—Arch of the Knees

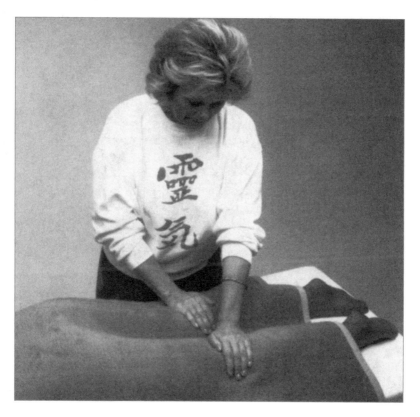

In the arch of the knees

B 9—Feet

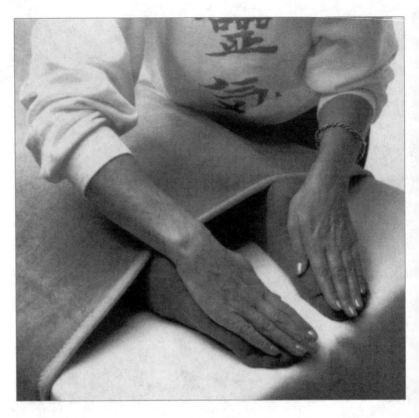

Bottom of the feet to get grounded. The fingertips touch the tips
of the toes (end position).

Special Position—Sciatica

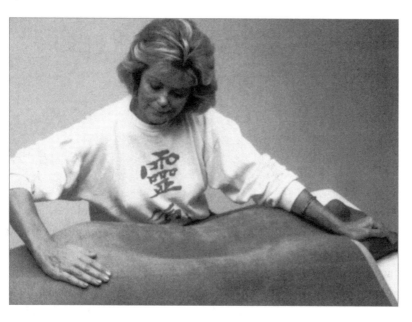

In case of sciatica pain, put one hand on the affected side of the buttocks, and the other on the heel of the foot of the same side. Also treat the entire leg from top to bottom.

12

FIRST AID WITH REIKI

It goes without saying that a medical doctor should always be called in cases of emergencies and accidents. But you can stay with an injured person, giving support and calmness with your Reiki hands until help arrives.

Because the injured person will in most cases be in shock, it is generally best to apply the hands onto the solar plexus or the adrenal gland. It is also a good idea to make a connection between the front and the back. In this case, one hand would be applied to the solar plexus and the other to the adrenal gland. This brings back the innate Healer and will ease the shock. Later the outer shoulders can be treated. If circumstances don't allow this sort of treatment, then apply one hand to the back of the head (medulla oblongata) and the other to the forehead (forehead chakra). Otherwise simply hold one or both of the person's hands—Reiki will always flow.

Those trained in First Aid should proceed with the necessary treatment. Reiki will automatically flow with this treatment, and the Reiki First Aid positions can be used in addition. We have given First Aid with Reiki on numerous occasions and have always been surprised and delighted by how wonderfully the injured person was able to calm down.

There can always be situations where you are in a remote area and there is no medical aid available (during trips into the wilderness, for instance). Here Reiki will always be ready to use, and it should be used repeatedly and for longer periods depending on how severe the injury is. In cases of poisoning through insects or snakebites, it will be necessary to give Reiki, with the appropriate emergency treatment, for several hours without interruption so the poison can be eliminated from the body.

Suggestions for First Aid with Reiki

- **Fear.** Hands on the solar plexus, adrenal glands, and the back of the head. Also mental treatment with the 2nd Degree.

- **Stroke.** Immediately call a physician. Until a physician arrives, apply hands to the upper and lower stomach, not directly to the heart.

- **Insect Bites.** Directly onto the bite for twenty to thirty minutes. No swelling will occur if Reiki is given immediately.

- **Broken bones.** Bones should be set by a doctor before Reiki is given. Hands can be applied directly onto the cast.

- **Bruises.** Immediately apply hands directly onto the bruise for twenty to thirty minutes.

- **Shock/Accident.** Immediately call a physician. Until the physician arrives, apply hands to the solar plexus and/or the adrenal glands. Later apply them to the outer shoulders.

- **Burns.** Apply Reiki to the injured area from a distance, for twenty to thirty minutes, possibly in intervals. Pain may increase at first, but will then recede. Blisters can be avoided if Reiki is given immediately.

- **Sprains.** Apply Reiki to the sprain for thirty to sixty minutes, depending on the degree of the sprain. Repeat several times.

- **Wounds.** Apply Reiki to the injury, perhaps in intervals. Later over the bandage.

Depending on the degree of injury, it is advisable to see a physician. Reiki will always support the positive aspect of any treatment and further healing.

13

SHORT REIKI TREATMENTS

The short Reiki treatment can be used anywhere, anytime, if someone does not feel well or is exhausted and in need of an energy charge. It is also very helpful in cases of stress and headaches. Let the Reiki receiver rest comfortably in a chair. Make sure the legs are not crossed or the hands folded, as this could block the energy flow.

Begin by placing your hands in the following positions:

1. First on the shoulders.

2. Then on the top of the head—do not touch the crown chakra directly—or on the sides of the head.

3. After this, put one hand on the medulla oblongata, and the other over the forehead.

4. Follow this by putting one hand on the 7th vertebra (the prominent), and the other on the throat.

5. Then put one hand on the sternum/heart-center (between the breasts) and the other on the back.

6. Follow this by putting one hand on the solar plexus (stomach), and the other on the back.

7. Finally, put one hand on the lower stomach, and the other on the back down to the tailbone.

A short Reiki treatment like this harmonizes the chakras as each area is touched consecutively.

14

Harmonizing the Chakras with Reiki

Harmonizing the chakras with Reiki is very effective. It can either be included in a complete treatment or can be done separately if there is not enough time for a complete treatment. You can accomplish a lot in only twenty minutes.

The chakras can be harmonized in various ways.

1. **The chakras are harmonized simultaneously.** Apply one hand on the 1st chakra (root chakra on the front of the body) and the other on the 6th chakra (forehead chakra). Feel the energy and wait until it is sensed in both chakras (usually the root chakra feels cold and the forehead chakra is hot), and both chakras feel the same temperature. Although not an actual temperature, it is the way the energy is perceived. Now proceed with the other chakras in the same way, following the 2nd chakra (spleen chakra) with the 5th chakra (throat chakra), then the 3rd chakra (solar plexus) with the 4th chakra (heart chakra). Because the chakras are in relation to each other—the 1st with the 6th, the 2nd with 5th, and the 3rd with the 4th—it is important to harmonize them. Let intuition be your guide. Variations are possible; for example, the 2nd chakra could need harmonizing with the 4th chakra. In cases of bladder problems, for instance, harmonize the 1st chakra with the

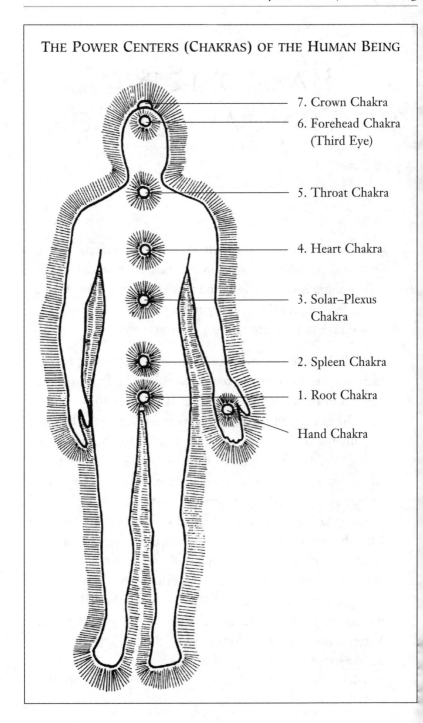

THE POWER CENTERS (CHAKRAS) OF THE HUMAN BEING

7. Crown Chakra

6. Forehead Chakra (Third Eye)

5. Throat Chakra

4. Heart Chakra

3. Solar–Plexus Chakra

2. Spleen Chakra

1. Root Chakra

Hand Chakra

6th chakra. The bladder-relating acupuncture points on the forehead also conduct the energy. The usual order is:

- 1st chakra with the 6th chakra.

- 2nd chakra with the 5th chakra.

- 3rd chakra with the 4th chakra or the 6th chakra.

- 1st chakra with the 4th chakra.

- 2nd chakra with the 4th chakra.

2. The chakras can also be harmonized or balanced by keeping one hand on the 1st or the 6th chakra while all other chakras are harmonized with it. This is done as follows: One hand is applied to the 1st chakra (root), the other to the 6th chakra (forehead). The hands stay in this position until the same energy is flowing in both. Then one hand is applied to the 5th chakra (throat), while the lower hand stays on the 1st (root) chakra. This is repeated with all the other chakras (4th, 3rd, 2nd chakras), and always until the same energy flows. If a person is very much *in their head*—which is almost always the case—it is best to start with the 6th chakra (forehead), then keep one hand there while all other chakras are consecutively harmonized with it. (Those who have received the Reiki initiation of the 2nd Degree can also reinforce the harmonizing, or balancing, with the corresponding symbols).

3. Short Reiki treatments (see Chapter 13) can also harmonize the chakras. The general rule is to let Reiki guide your intuition. This may lead you to even more possibilities.

Chakra Harmonizing (Self-Treatment)

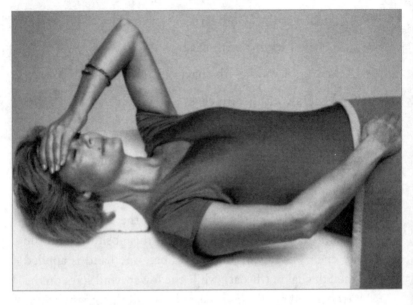

Balancing the Root Chakra (1) with the Forehead Chakra (6).

Chakra Harmonizing (Self-Treatment)

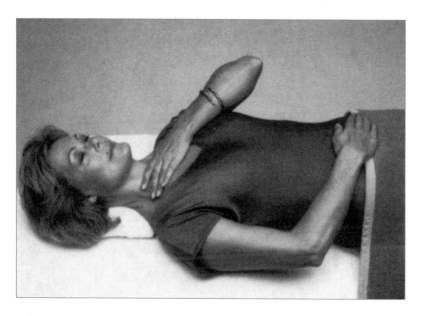

Balancing the Spleen Chakra (2) with the Throat Chakra (5).

Chakra Harmonizing (Self-Treatment)

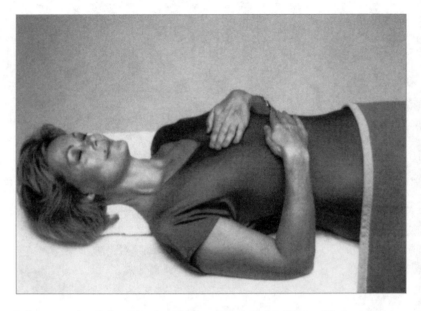

Balancing the Solar Plexus Chakra (3) with the Heart Chakra (4).

Chakra Harmonizing (Treating Others)

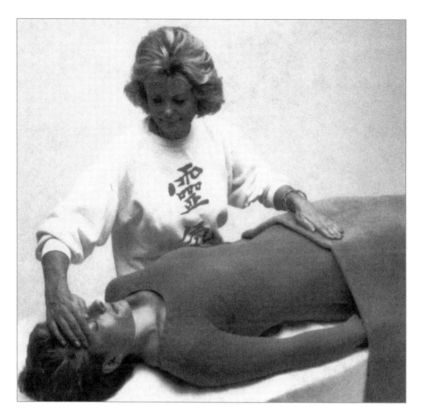

Balancing the Root Chakra (1) with the Forehead Chakra (6).

Chakra Harmonizing (Treating Others)

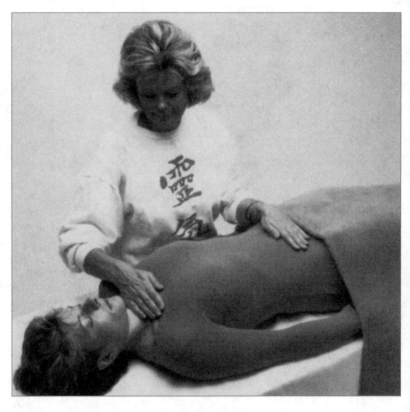

Balancing the Spleen Chakra (2) with the Throat Chakra (5).

Chakra Harmonizing (Treating Others)

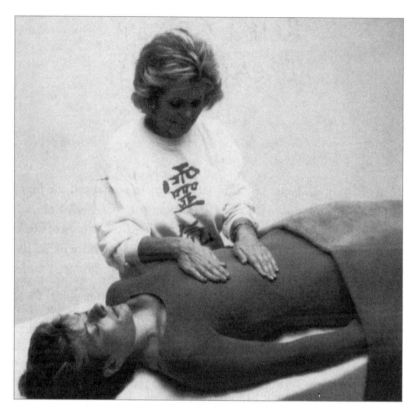

Balancing the Solar Plexus Chakra (3) with the Heart Chakra (4).

15

Reiki Group Treatments

I n meetings of Reiki practitioners, the main point, and the high-light, is often a Reiki Group Treatment for everybody.

In group treatments, one person is treated by a group of Reiki practitioners in this manner: The group decides who will be the first to receive a treatment, and this chosen person lies on a table, while the others place themselves around the table. A good way to begin is for all the Reiki givers to form a circle around the receiver; they hold hands to attune themselves before the treatment begins, and then everyone finds a place for their hands.

We recommend applying the hands as follows:

- One person touches the head.

- Several people touch the organs on the front of the body.

- One person touches the insides of the thighs (if appropriate).

- One person touches the knees.

- One person touches the feet.

It is a good idea to ask the receiver if the touch is comfortable (hands should be applied without pressure), and if there is a place which needs to be specially treated.

While the receiver is being turned to the other side, it is best to keep the hands in contact with the body, to allow the person to glide into the new position on the back.

When a lot of people are in the group, a second or third group can be formed to accommodate all in turn. Those who cannot find a spot directly connected to the receiver can put their hands onto the shoulders of the others and can form an outer circle around the group treating the receiver.

This type of group treatment has been used often and is always a wonderful experience for everyone present. Reiki energy is multiplied through the group—it should be noted here that the power of the group's energy can sometimes lead to emotional reactions.

For a balanced process, the following details should be taken into account:

- Everyone present should have a turn at receiving a group treatment during the meeting.

- The room should be aired out before every treatment.

- A quiet environment should be created (no doorbell or phone).

- Conversations should be avoided during the treatment.

- The receiver should rest comfortably.

- Quiet, meditative music supports the treatment.

- Choose a person for each treatment who will begin by smoothing the aura, will watch the agreed-upon time for the treatment, and in conclusion will smooth the aura once more.

A group treatment, with six to eight people treating, will usually run ten minutes each for the front and the back of the Reiki receiver, about twenty minutes total. If the receiver is in an emotional state (for example, crying or laughing) at the end of the session, then the treatment should be continued until the receiver is harmonized.

16

REIKI TREATMENTS FOR EXPECTANT MOTHERS AND BABIES

Reiki has a very positive impact on a mother and baby if regular treatments (perhaps once a week) are started during the first months of pregnancy when morning sickness, depression, or other discomforts of these first months can be eased.

During a Reiki treatment of the mother, the child will begin to kick and move inside the womb, as if the child is happy, but after a while it will calm down as mother and child are in harmony. If the mother has received Reiki initiation, she can treat herself and her womb—through this process, many strong babies, charged with energy, have been born. The mother should not, however, participate in a Reiki workshop later than the beginning of the seventh month of her pregnancy.

After the birth, the mother can treat her baby with Reiki, especially its feet, as that will help overcome the shock of birth more quickly. In any case, Reiki is always flowing, as when the mother is stroking her child or holding it in her arms. Reiki can also help with any complications the child may have. For instance, a three-year-old girl ran crying to her mother after she fell and hurt herself, saying, "Mommy, please put your big hot Reiki hand on my arm."

There are also cases where Reiki supports fertility. A woman who was unable to get pregnant for ten years finally became pregnant after her 1st Degree Reiki workshop. In another case, a fifty-year-old man, who had previously tried to father a child, finally had success after the workshop. In both cases, wonderful babies were born.

Should the mother have health problems during her pregnancy, or perhaps even run the risk of losing the child, Reiki, in tandem with the efforts of the treating doctor, can be very supportive.

17

REIKI FOR THE DYING

Reiki can be helpful when working with the very ill, infirm, or dying, as well as with their caretakers in hospitals or nursing homes. The caretakers are always able to recharge themselves with Reiki while they do their work, and this is an important prerequisite to being able to help others.

The uses of Reiki in these situations are countless. Beginning with holding a needy person's hand if they are afraid, or applying a hand on the person's shoulders, Reiki will flow with every contact, and ideally a complete treatment can be given.

Reiki can be very calming and will help people and animals during the death process. It will let the natural process of dying take place, because Reiki is an intelligent force and follows the course of life.

The hand of the dying person can be held, or a treatment can be given to ease complications. This dying person will feel protected, and it will be easier to let go into the next dimension. Death in its literal sense doesn't exist. Birth and death are a transformation into a different form of being. The physical level is left behind. The soul, or our immortal essence, has slipped into a body during our lifetime on earth and will leave this body during the process of dying. "Dying is only a move into a prettier house" said the well-known researcher Dr. Elizabeth Kübler-Ross in her book, *On Life after Death*.

Selected Experiences

Here are stories from those who used Reiki in the care of the elderly, or accompanying people on their dying journey.

Volunteering with Reiki

"In the course of our volunteer work with the elderly, we visit many hospitals, nursing, and caretaking homes. Often the poor people we meet are just miserable and confused, needing a helping hand. We have observed that when we let go of a person's hand, the other hand will spontaneously be taken, and the energy will flow. This, for us, is a beautiful miracle which we are thankful to experience." (*Petra and Ernst*)

Reiki Relief in Last-Stage Cancer

"My wife was suffering from cancer in its last stage. Traditional medical practices did not see any more practical options for treatment. Because of this, I decided to give up my skeptical academic attitude toward things outside the scientific framework. I attended the next available Reiki workshop and received the 1st Degree.

"During the workshop, my initial attitude melted like snow in the sun of spring. Already, things were happening that I never thought were possible. Even the first shy attempts to help my wife during the workshop resulted in her feeling better and she told me, 'I Think you are able to heal.' At the end of the workshop, many of the other participants wished me luck for my difficult voyage. There also were some there who had experienced cancer with members of their own families. They warned me to be modest in my expectations, and to expect more of a relief from the complications than an actual cure.

"However, my optimistic and energetic nature steered me toward healing. I immediately began giving Reiki at home over four consecutive days, and then in two-day, and later three-day intervals. My wife felt better every time, and I realized what incredible amounts of energy were flowing in certain places. I was aware of what this meant. There were signs of hope, such as places I had not touched, although my wife said that I had, where all the pain had disappeared. There were also discouraging signs, much like extinguished candles that could have burned much longer.

"When my wife could not lie down anymore, I gave her Reiki sitting up. It was impossible to maintain the regular positions, and I was forced to follow my own feelings and develop new positions. When the touch of my hands led to discomfort and even pain, I learned to work with the aura and got the same results as if I had applied my hands. I had my wife tell me at what point the power of my hands became uncomfortable, and made a note of how my hands felt to me at this distance. Without further instructions from her, my wife was surprised when I was able to keep the right distance, which was quite different at different parts of the body.

"Metastasis in her lung caused strong cough-attacks, especially while driving in a cold car. Simply extending my hand to the front of her chest was enough to stop the attack, and she would be free from coughing for half an hour. We called it the *cough candy*. When her lung began to slowly fill with water, the coughing caused her to have great trouble lying down and trying to fall asleep. I would greet her in bed with my extended hands, and immediately put one hand on the fear point at the back of the head (position H 3) and the other hand in the middle of the back, roughly in position B 3, and she would fall asleep within five minutes. When this happened the first time, she told me it was a miracle. She had never fallen asleep so fast, and she had never slept through the night so well. We kept up this routine until the end.

"We were both trained in meditation through yoga, books, and other workshops. We used meditation in such a way that my wife would try to reach complete stillness. Later we would both meditate before a Reiki treatment, and I would return from my state of meditation earlier than my wife and then give her Reiki.

"We meditated long and deeply on the last evening we were

granted together. It was especially beautiful because, as it turned out later, a Reiki friend was giving us distant Reiki at the same time. With Reiki, I had finally found the strength to say yes to the Father's request, *Thy will be done.* Until that day I had always had great difficulty with this request. Now Reiki's blessing stood behind my wife and I prayed humbly: 'Where I cannot heal, let me help. Where I cannot help, let me ease.' We do not give Reiki against God's will, but because of His divine grace.

"We did not succeed in curing the cancer. My wife died peacefully and quietly the following night. She escaped a much more terrible fate, as she had been threatened with a slow and painful death through suffocation, but she passed away in a quiet, fearless way and had no struggle before death. Instead, she smiled in her death. This is where the calming quality of Reiki is documented.

"After my wife died, there were some people who told me that I had not helped with Reiki. But I know that I helped my wife on her difficult path. It really depends how it is viewed. A glass of water can be half empty or half full. It is the same with the physical condition. At this point I would like to thank everyone who gave me the strength with distant Reiki to make it through those hard times. I would also like to thank all those who cared for my wife, be it with or without Reiki." (*Peter*)

Calming Effects of Reiki Healing

"When we arrived in England last spring, my girlfriend's mother was dying. She was constantly vomiting and choking, and was very nervous. I was alone with her and gave her Reiki for a few minutes. When my girlfriend returned, she was surprised at how quiet her mother had become. She had stopped vomiting and was resting in her bed. After I left, I gave her distant Reiki for one or two days and she died very peacefully on the fifth day. I also came across difficulties, and at times the light seemed to be far away. However, I believe that I am also on the way to trusting Reiki, the divine love, 100 percent." (*Birgit*)

Reiki Testimonials for Dying Animals

It is also possible to accompany animals in their dying process. We have had this experience ourselves with our dogs. We touched them with our hands and held them after they were put to sleep. We also helped them on their way by using distant Reiki.

This should encourage all animal lovers to be with their pets in the dying process—for example while the pet is being put to sleep by a veterinarian. This is the last rite you can give a faithful companion.

A Reiki Friend's Report on a Much-Loved Dying Animal

"A friend recommended Reiki when I told her about my cancer-stricken dog. I went to a Reiki workshop to help the dog, who meant a lot to me. I was in despair because I knew he would die soon. I prayed to God and was not ready to lose him. On the first evening of the workshop, I gained what could perhaps be called a deeper comprehension, and in the course of the workshop, I experienced a wonderful development. I didn't realize how much I had matured until I returned home. My dog couldn't greet me anymore; he was lying apathetically on his side. My mother told me this had only occurred in the last few hours. I treated my dog with Reiki for an hour, which he seemed to enjoy. When someone rang the doorbell, he jumped up, barked, and wagged his tail to greet the visitor. Even though she is very critical, my mother was completely astonished. Then came the day when I had to let my dog go. This day, which I had feared for years, went by harmoniously. Although I was not able to let go of my dog's physical shell without sadness—I am not that far yet—I was able to let go of him with only good thoughts. Today I think this dog had fulfilled his task on earth by connecting me with Reiki. Although I now have another dog, I think that my first one was a special creature." (*Karin*)

18

REIKI TREATMENT FOR ANIMALS

Animals like Reiki a lot, especially our dogs, cats, guinea pigs, hamsters, and birds, but also horses, cows, chickens, sheep, and pigs. Sick animals will like getting Reiki. Animals are not disrupted by their intellect; they gratefully take in the energy and immediately feel that something special is coming from Reiki hands.

When treating animals, be aware how they turn toward your hands. Animals usually show exactly where they want the Reiki hands placed. If you move your hands, you can observe that the animal will turn itself in such a way that your hands touch the original places. The animal will also stay still as long as it needs Reiki, which will depend on how sick the animal is. Usually you can treat an animal for twenty to thirty minutes. Dogs stay still longer, while cats are very sensitive to energy and will jump away earlier. Very sick animals can be treated for one or two hours. They will let you know when to stop, either by jumping away or standing up.

When the pictures for this book were taken, the cat Maria Theresa was very sick. She had a cold, a sore throat, and was breathing heavily. Brigitte applied her hands for an hour, and then, feeling much better, the cat rolled and stretched itself. Her owner later told us the cat had another attack the next day and was breathing heavily for about twenty minutes, but after she gave her Reiki, the attack was over within twenty minutes. Twenty-four hours later, it was clear that Maria Theresa felt better because she ate and drank for the first time in seven days. In cases like this, it is advantageous to treat the animal every day for a period of time.

It is also a good idea to treat the organs that are connected to a given illness. For example, the spleen (immune system), kidneys (secretion), and head/throat, in case of a cold. It is exactly the same as in humans. And, after surgery on an animal, long, daily Reiki treatments can accelerate the healing process.

There are many opportunities to help animals with Reiki, and it can be very supportive for veterinarians, animal activists, and animal homes. Because Reiki affects body, spirit, and soul, it is also very beneficial for animals that have behavior problems or show signs of abuse. Abused dogs and cats don't usually want to be touched at first, but later, when they feel Reiki's radiation, they calm down quickly. It can also be helpful to pet them and talk to them. An animal's psyche reacts positively to Reiki, and often animals will lick the hands of a stranger who is giving them Reiki.

During workshops, participants often say that their animals behave completely differently after they return home. We have heard of dogs that were surprised, sniffed excitedly, and sometimes ran away. After a while they come back, want a lot of love, and act frisky. Sometimes they will show completely opposite behavior. A dog that was not very accessible before became very friendly. We have similar reports about cats. In the first night after the Reiki initiation, some will lie on their owner's stomach or another body part, and even come into the bed although they may never have done so before.

If you are treating a larger animal, such as a horse or a cow, your hands can be applied right on the affected body parts; for example, a lame or swollen leg can be treated directly. If the leg is bandaged, put your hands over the bandage, Reiki will go through. This is also recommended on the head and behind the ears. Horses will usually let their head hang in a relaxed way and begin to doze off (as seen in the pictures). The horse in the pictures is called Godiva and is ridden by Brigitte.

Distant Reiki treatments (2nd Degree) can be used with large animals living in the wild, or with animals in a zoo. When we saw some whales in trouble on TV, we gave them distant Reiki.

While we were in the stable taking pictures of the horse, we saw a small kitty playing with the butterfly in the picture that was hurt and unable to fly. Brigitte took it in her hand and gave it Reiki. Completely paralyzed at first, it began to move and we put it in a nearby bush to recuperate and fly off. It is also possible to breathe new life into birds that fly against a glass window. Brigitte once found a small hedgehog that had fallen into the drain of a swimming pool and was completely exhausted; but after twenty minutes of Reiki, it began to move and cruised into the garden.

We have a special place in our hearts for animals. We have both had dogs and have had many opportunities to help them with Reiki.

The Best Way to Treat Animals

Cats and Dogs

Behind the ears, one hand on the head the other under the throat; onto the chest, stomach, back, hips, and the organs. Treat the pain areas, such as a wounded paw, directly.

Horses and Cows

Treat on the head, behind the ears, as you do cats and dogs, and in the middle over the eyes. Also treat a horse's lame legs over the bandages.

Fish

Put your hands on the fish tank.

Birds

Hold the bird in your hand, or put your hands on the cage.

Animals in a Zoo and Those in Emergencies or Catastrophes

If possible, treat the animal directly, otherwise give distant Reiki (2nd Degree).

Reiki Treatment of Animals

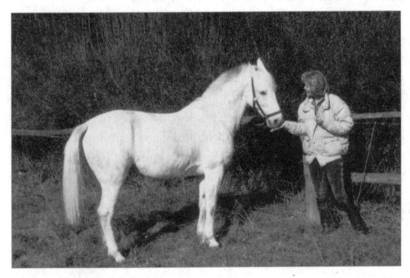

Godiva, a sixteen-year-old mare.

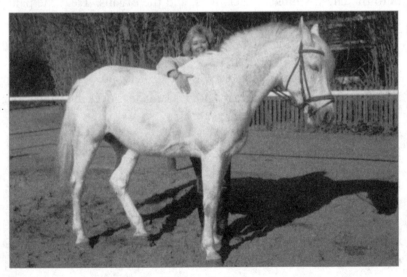

Godiva is completely relaxed when Reiki flows.

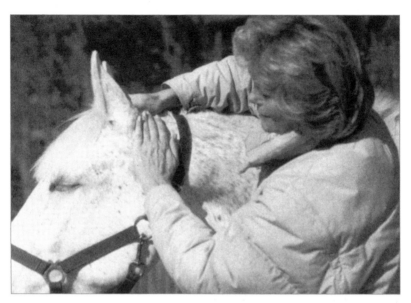

Godiva especially likes Reiki behind the ears. She is almost asleep.

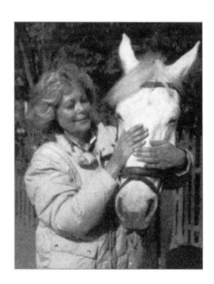

This is the position for treating a cold. Godiva is very relaxed.

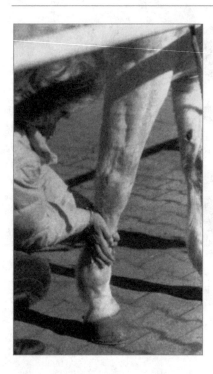

When the horse's legs have a problem, we hold them with our hands. This also works over a bandage.

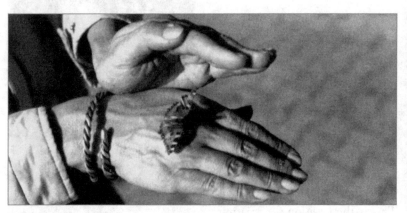

This is the butterfly we treated with Reiki in the stable.

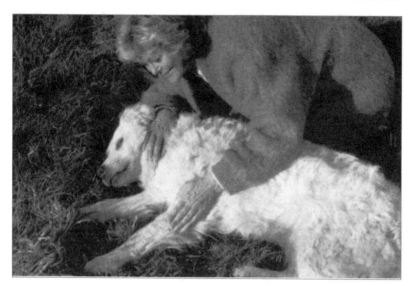

Danuta, a thirteen-year-old Kuvasz dog, enjoys receiving Reiki very much. This position works well for arthritis in the joints.

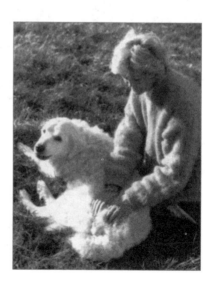

For problems in the hips, this is how to apply the hands.

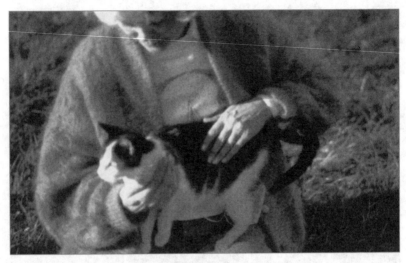

Reiki treatment for chest and kidneys.

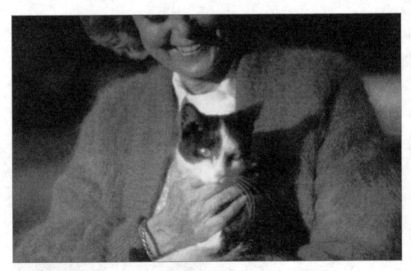

Maria Theresa got Reiki on her chest for her cold.

19

REIKI TREATMENT OF PLANTS, MINERALS, AND OBJECTS

B ecause Reiki is an energy that makes all life on earth grow and
thrive, the results of Reiki treatments are especially visible in
plants.

Here is a way to test this:

Plant some sprouts and treat half of them daily with Reiki,
while letting the other half grow naturally, without Reiki. You
will find that the Reiki treatments yield stronger sprouts.

When planting seeds, hold the grains in your hands for a while
before you plant them. Give them Reiki every day while they
sprout.

With young plants, simply hold them by their roots for several minutes.

With potted plants, hold your hands around the pot and treat
the roots. If necessary you can also treat the leaves.

With cut flowers, hold the stems for several minutes, and later
put your hands around the vase.

You can also treat your garden from a distance with 2nd Degree
Reiki. We have heard about a garden that was treated with Reiki
from a distance and yielded a rich harvest of fruit while all the other
gardens in the area had a terrible harvest.

Forests, especially, can be helped with distant Reiki healing. And when you have a chance to be in a forest, you can hug a tree.

Minerals, such as crystals, precious stones, and jewelry, can be cleaned or charged with Reiki energy. Simply hold these kinds of objects under running water for a short time and then hold them in your hands. Since matter is condensed vibration or spirit, it can be permeated by Reiki's energy.

From personal experiences and from numerous reports received over the years, it has been observed that:

- Car batteries can be recharged (please be sure to use gloves when touching the battery, or give distant Reiki).

- The ignition system of a car was repaired.

- Jammed locks were opened.

- Vibrations in a room can be substantially improved or changed.

Sometimes situations are difficult to analyze, but remember, it is always a good idea to try Reiki.

20

USING REIKI
FOR FOOD AND DRINK

You can also give Reiki to the food that's eaten and drunk. Reiki really acts as a spiritual blessing of food, so it will be enriched with universal life energy. Since all matter has a certain vibrational frequency, it is possible to increase this frequency through Reiki. For example, if you eat in restaurants a lot, you can change the vibrations of the food if necessary (it's possible the cook was in a bad mood, in which case that vibration would be in the food). Hold your hands inconspicuously over the food and drink, and this will allow you to digest the meal better. It is also possible to apply your hands to your stomach afterwards.

When preparing meals at home, you can also give your food Reiki. Working with your (washed) hands as much as possible, use them to knead dough or batter for bread and cakes, or mix a salad. Everything that is touched with Reiki hands will receive this energy.

It has been reported that the taste of water or other drinks changes considerably after being treated with Reiki. This may be a good idea for an experiment.

Sprouts and seedlings which receive daily Reiki treatments will sprout much faster than those that don't. Try this yourself. Reiki improves the quality and nutritional value of foods and drinks.

Pizza Parlor Reiki

This story from a workshop participant who owns a pizzeria shows how the everyday uses of Reiki are limitless.

"I was busy making a pizza in my restaurant, when I suddenly thought about my wife who was attending a Reiki workshop with Horst. Somehow I was overcome with the idea that I should make a Reiki pizza. I got into the right mood, treated the dough with Reiki, and gave the whole pizza Reiki before I put it into the oven, then again before I served it.

"When my guest—a regular customer—had finished eating, I went to his table to take the plate and asked, as I always do, if he liked the pizza.

" 'Yes' he said, 'but do you have a new cook?'

" 'No,' I replied.

" 'Did you maybe use a new recipe for the dough?'

"Again I said no, and asked, 'Didn't you like it?' "

" 'Oh yes I did,' said my customer, 'it was exceptionally good.'

"He seemed a bit irritated and shook his head. 'If the cook and the dough are the same . . . , this pizza was good, exceptionally good . . . I mean, I always like the food here . . . but this pizza, I don't know . . . this pizza was somehow different.' " (*Enrico*)

21

Long Distance Reiki
of the 2nd Degree

Chapter 4, "How to Become a Reiki Channel," explains the circumstances under which a person can receive the 2nd Degree, and how it is different from the 1st Degree. An important aspect of the 2nd Degree is the ability to heal from a distance. It also makes it possible to transmit positive spiritual messages to reinforce the healing power.

The symbols that become familiar in the 2nd Degree initiation allow you the giver to connect with the person you are treating on a mental and spiritual level. In the same way it is possible to connect with divine power, beyond space and time.

You can also give *yourself* a distant treatment. This way the higher self will treat the body, spirit, and soul of you. You will see yourself from a higher place. You can also treat your back, and can influence and change your thoughts in a positive direction through a mental transmission.

This process will transmit loving, healing energy over a bridge of light.

Please understand there can be no further discussion of distant treatments at this point because that occurs only as part of the 2nd Degree initiation.

22

THE UNIVERSAL RULE OF
GIVING AND RECEIVING

For every Reiki treatment given, an exchange of energy should take place. By *exchange of energy* we mean that something should be given for the treatment received.

If both people have been initiated into Reiki, the simplest way for this to happen would be to exchange treatments. If this is not the case, then a donation of money, gifts, flowers, theater tickets, or trading other types of work can serve as an exchange of energy for the treatment.

It is not the Reiki energy that is paid for or traded, but the time which the Reiki-giving person has made accessible. Since this person could have spent the time working for his or her livelihood, some kind of reimbursement should be forthcoming. If the practitioner does not want money for personal use, then consider making a donation to a charity or a community organization. In any case, those giving treatment professionally with Reiki will need to be reimbursed for their time and they will charge a certain fee.

If the giver is not willing to receive something for a treatment, then it might be necessary to get in touch with her or his inner self to see if there is a problem with receiving, or with self-esteem. It could also be that this awakens feelings of commitment or guilt in the receiver, or even turns that person into the beggar (see Chapter 2 for Dr. Usui's treatment of beggars). Whatever the situation, the client should be given the chance to pay for treatment to be freed from the weight of commitments and karmic responsibilities.

However, if someone wants to consume only, and does not want to give something for a treatment, then it could be that this person is not actively involved in the healing process, or the Reiki practitioner has a personal problem with receiving him/herself. That is why the kind and amount of the energy exchange should be discussed clearly before beginning a series of treatments.

The Universal Rule of Giving and Receiving is in relation to the natural principle of resonance. There is much truth in old proverbs, for example:

"As above—so below."

"You reap what you sow."

"Do unto others as you would have them do unto you."

In accordance with spiritual rules, an exchange of energy has to take place in order to keep harmony in the universe. As lesson number 108 from the *Course in Miracles* states:

"To give and to receive are one in truth."

Another example clarifies this: someone not willing to receive will disrupt the flow of energy, which is exactly the same as if one refuses to give. The cycle of energy has to be kept alive!

Life is a constant process of giving and receiving. After all, our life on this planet is a gift—and we are able to give so much. It is a constant allowing of the flow. Wherever there is flow or movement, there is life.

GLOBAL PEACE ON EARTH THROUGH REIKI

Peace begins with you. Peace of the soul is a personal matter. It has to start with your own inner thoughts and be extended outward. It is your inner peace that will create a peaceful world. With Reiki, you can feel your inner peace and be in harmony with all other living beings.

Here are some peace activities in which you can participate.

For All Friends of Reiki

Every Sunday from 9:00 to 9:15 AM, Pacific Time.

Peace Clock, 12 Noon

Begin wherever you are, for one minute every day at 12:00 noon, place yourself in deep, quiet meditation for worldwide peace. The goal is that, on January 1, every human being on earth will take part in this meditation. For further information:

Peace Clock
P.O. Box 8307
Calabasas, CA 91302, USA

Global Healing Meditation

Annually on December 31st at 12 noon Greenwich Time, and on the last day of every month, place yourself in deep, quiet meditation for global healing. For more information:

The Planetary Commission for Global Healing
c/o The Quartus Foundation
P.O. Box 1768
Boerne TX 78006, USA
Telephone: (830) 249-3985

The Planetary Commission is calling upon everyone to get together in thoughts during those days for a worldwide healing meditation. The first time this meditation took place was on December 31, 1986, and more than 41 million people participated.

These numbers grew as the event continued in 1987, 1988, 1989, and each year after that. More information is available in the book, *The Planetary Commission*, by John Randolph Price.

International Healing Meditation—
John Randolph Price

In the beginning—
In the beginning God.
In the Beginning, God created heaven and earth.
And God said, let there be light; and there was light.

Now it is time for the new beginning.
I am a co-creator with God, and it is a new Heaven that
    comes,
as the Good Will of God is expressed on Earth through me.
It is the kingdom of Light, Love, Peace, and Understanding.
And I am doing my part to reveal its Reality.
I begin with me.
I am a living soul and the Spirit of God dwells in me, as me.
I and the Father are one, and all that the Father has is
    mine.
In Truth, I am the Christ of God.

What is true of me is true of everyone,
for God is all and all is God.
I see only the Spirit of God in every Soul.
And to every man, woman, and child on earth I say:
I love you, for you are me.
You are my Holy Self.

I now open my heart,
and let the pure essence of Unconditional Love pour out.
I see it as a Golden Light radiating from the center of
    my being,
and I feel its Divine Vibration in and through me, above
    and below me.

I am one with the Light.
I am filled with the Light.
I am illumined by the Light.
I am the Light of the world.

With purpose of mind, I send forth the Light
I let the radiance go before me to join the other Lights.
I know this is happening all over the world at this moment.
I see the merging Lights.
There is now one Light. We are the Light of the World.

The one Light of Love, Peace, and Understanding is
    moving.
It flows across the face of the Earth,
touching and illuminating every soul in the shadow of the
    illusion.
And where there was darkness, there is now the Light of
    Reality.
And the Radiance grows, permeating, saturating every
    form of life.
There is only the vibration of one Perfect Life now.
All the kingdoms of the earth respond,
and the planet is alive with Light and Love.

There is total Oneness
and in this Oneness we speak the word.
Let the sense of separation by dissolved.
Let mankind be returned to Godkind.

Let peace come forth in every mind.
Let Love flow forth from every heart.
Let forgiveness reign in every soul
Let understanding be the common bond.

And now from the Light of the world,
the One Presence and Power of the Universe responds.
The Activity of God is healing and harmonizing
    Planet Earth.
Omnipotence is made manifest.

I am seeing the salvation of the planet before my very eyes,
as all false beliefs and error patterns are dissolved.
The sense of separation is no more; the healing has
    taken place,
and the world is restored to sanity.

This is the beginning of Peace on Earth and Good Will
    toward all,
as Love flows forth from every heart,
forgiveness reigns in every soul,
and all hearts and minds are one in perfect understanding.

It is done. And it is so.

23

REIKI POSITIONS FOR ENHANCING HEALTH

Reiki treatments can support any therapeutic treatment. It is, however, important to once again point out that a physician should always be consulted before the Reiki treatment of an illness.

It is also always recommended to give a whole treatment, and follow it up with concentrated treatments in the special positions for certain ailments, which are explained below. In case of emergencies or accidents, please refer to Chapter 12 on First Aid with Reiki.

Head Position = H

Basic Position = BP

Back Position = B

Accident. As described under "Shock to the Spine" and "Trauma:" B 3, B 4, adrenal glands, and solar plexus; BP 3 in case of bleeding, hold directly over the affected area.

AIDS. *Treat every day*, especially H 2A, H 2B, H 3, and H 5, BP 1, and BP 2, especially spleen; BP 4, BP 5, B 3, and B 4 kidneys.

Allergies. Sinus H 1, H 3, B 3, and B 4, adrenal glands, kidneys.

Amnesia. H 4 and ovaries, BP 4 and prostate, B 7.

Amputation. Treat the limb for blood circulation. In case of pain treat as described under Pain. Later put on the prosthesis and treat the bottom of both feet or the limb as if it were in place.

Anemia. Spleen, BP 2, left side, liver BP 1, from the side onto the head.

Arthritis. Directly on the affected spots, such as front and back of the knee, B 3, B 4, kidneys.

BP, R, especially kidneys, affected areas. Treat as described under Pain. Sciatica positions in case the lower limbs are affected.

Asthma. BP 5, also directly under the chest, collarbone. H 1, over sinus (lightly press a finger onto the sides of the nose bone).

Athlete's foot. BP and feet.

Back problems. BP, especially BP 3, BP 4, BP 5; B 1–B 7, areas of pain.

Balance. BP 1 (gallbladder) and on the side of the head.

Birth. BP, especially BP 3, BP 4, BP 5, B, especially lower back. This will help open the pelvis, through which the baby attains a good position for a painless birth.

Bladder. In general: BP 4, V position, bladder, and B 3, B 4, kidneys, H 1, H 4.

Urine Condition: BP 1 and BP 2, BP 4, H 1.

Bleeding. BP 2, spleen, H, onto the head from the side.

Menstrual Bleeding. BP 2, BP 3 and BP 4, H, onto the side of the head.

Blood pressure, high. H 5, 15–20 minutes on the side of the throat, B 3 and B 4 over the kidneys and adrenal glands, under the armpits.

Breast tumor. BP, especially BP 4—15–20 minutes, BP 5 for some time, then over the tumor for 15–20 minutes, BP 2.

Breathing. BP 5, chest, underneath the breasts and shoulder/collarbone. H 1, slightly press the sides of the nose bone; B 2 and B 3 over the shoulder blades and over lower ribs to the right and left of the vertebrae. Feet, especially under the big toe.

Broken bones. Let the bone be set first, then directly on the broken spot (Reiki will go through plaster casts).

Bronchitis. BP 5, ribs directly underneath the chest and over the collarbone, H 1, press the sides of the nose, B 2, B 3, B 4.

Bursitis. In general: BP, H, B 3, and B 4, over the kidneys.

In the arms, neck, shoulder or chest:
Front: Shoulders at the end of the collarbone near the throat.
Back: B 1A, neck, shoulders.

In the arms, legs, or hips: B, next to the vertebrae and above the shoulder blades, both sides.

Burns. Acute: Directly over the burn, as close as possible.

Not acute: BP and over burn.

Cancer. BP 1, BP 2, BP 3, BP 4, BP 5; all positions are important, solar plexus and over the area of the tumor.

Tongue Cancer: Under the feet.

Breast Cancer: BP 4 and BP 5 for a longer period of time, then over the tumor.

Circulation. BP, especially BP 4, top of the shoulders, over the chest, above the nipples, rib cage, under the armpits, inner side of the thighs, H, on the side of the head.

Colds. BP, especially BP 5, BP 2, spleen, H 1, H 2B, H 3, also underneath the corners of the mouth (in case of throat pains, H 5).

Constipation. BP, especially BP 3, BP 5, also simultaneously one hand over the navel and the other under the neck.

Cough. BP, BP 5, H 1, H 5, throat, B 1–B 4.

Cramps. BP, especially BP 4, B lower back, B 5–B 7.

Depression. BP, H, especially H 3 and H 4, and B, especially B 3 and B 4, BP 5, collarbone.

Diabetes. BP, especially BP 1 (15 minutes), BP 2, and BP 3, over the navel, H, especially H 3, B 1, B 1A, B 2, B 3, especially in the neck on both sides of the vertebrae and B 7. Also the tip of the elbow, front of the shin bone, directly underneath the knee, pleura.

Digestion problems. See **Stomach.**

Dizziness. See **Balance.**

Ear. Injured Eardrum: Middle finger into the ear opening, the others onto the head for 15–20 minutes; H 2B and behind the ears.

Ear Pains: H 2B and BP 5.

Deafness: Treat like ear pains.

Eczema. BP, B, especially B 3 and B 4, kidneys, and lungs.

Emotional upset. BP, especially BP 3 solar plexus, and BP 4, BP 5, to the sides of the chest and in the line of the nipples, collarbone, H 2, from the side of the head, B, B 1, B 1A, B 2, B 3, and B 4.

Emphysema. BP, especially BP 5, collarbone, chest, back, throat, and pleura.

Energy deficiency. BP 3 (over navel and Hara), B, B 7, and H 4, short Reiki treatment.

Enuresis (Bedwetting). BP, especially over the bladder (20 minutes), B 3 and B 4 over the kidneys and lower back, B 7.

Eyes. For all eye problems: BP, especially BP 4 (for women), H 1— slightly press the fingers into the inner corner of the eye, against the eyeball and surface of the eye, also onto H 2A and H 3.

Cataract, cloudiness: Treat as above, 10 minutes in each position every day.

Squint eyes: BP, especially BP 4, as above.

Green cataract: As above, especially ovaries, also H 2A and BP for 10 minutes (slightly press the tips of the fingers behind the jawbone directly behind the ear), H 3.

Chalazion eye sore: BP and H, especially H 1 and temples, back, and especially kidneys.

Fasting. When hunger sets in: BP 3, BP 4, H 5, thyroid gland, B 3, B 4, and B 7.

Fever. BP, especially BP 5, H, especially H 1 and H 3, slightly press fingers along the cheekbones, especially BP 1, BP 2, B 3, B 4.

Flatulence. BP 1 and BP 2, BP 3, H 4.

Flu. BP, especially chest and breathing system, BP 1, liver, BP 2, spleen, BP 5; H under the chin, H 1, H 3, B 1–B 4, B over and between the shoulder blades, under the feet, especially the big toes.

Glaucoma. See **Eyes.**

Gout. Directly onto the affected spot, for example the knee, finger, or hand, BP 3.

Hair loss. BP, especially BP 4, B 3, B 4, kidneys, and adrenal glands.

Hay fever. H 1, H 3, B 3, B 4, kidneys, and adrenal glands, 20 minutes daily.

Headaches. BP, especially BP 1, BP 3, and BP 4, H, especially H 1, H 2A, H 2B, H 3, H 4, B especially upper vertebrae, shoulder area, B 1, B 1A, B 2A, B 3, B 7.

Heart. Cardiac Infarction: Call a doctor immediately; upper and lower stomach, kidneys.

Angina Pectoris: Especially BP 1, BP 2, BP 3, treat the diaphragm and body, thyroid gland, H, especially H 2, B 1–B 4, especially upper back and adrenal glands.

Stroke: Upper and lower stomach, kidneys, BP 1, BP 2, BP 3, B 3, and B 4.

Cramp: BP, especially BP 5, under the chest, above the nipples, rib cage under the arms, H 2–H 4.

Enlargement: BP, chest above the nipples, H, especially H 2.

Pounding: BP, especially navel, thyroid gland.

Heartburn. See **Stomach**.

Heat. BP, especially BP 4.

Hemorrhoids. B 7, over rectum (20 minutes), BP 2, spleen (15–20 minutes).

Hiccups. Arms over the head, treat the diaphragm and the body.

Hyperactivity. BP, especially BP 1 and BP 3, H 2A, H 3, on the side of the head.

Hypoglycemia. BP 1, (15–20 minutes), B over kidneys, tip of the elbows.

Infections. For infections of all kinds. Under the feet, especially in the middle of the foot, underneath the heel, also directly over the infection, BP 1, BP 2, BP 5, B 3, and B 4.

Injuries. Directly onto or over the injured area.

Kidneys. BP, especially BP 1, BP 2, BP 4, BP 5; H, H 2B; B 3, and B 4, collarbone.

Knee. BP, BP 4, especially groin area, greater trochanter B, especially kidneys, kneecap, and inner side of the knee.

Larynx. Over the throat.

Legs. In general: BP, groin area, and greater trochanter.

Blood circulation: BP, especially BP 4, H 4, inner thighs.

Swollen Legs: BP, H 4, B 3, and B4, kidneys.

Pain in the legs: BP, especially BP 4 (very important) also greater trochanter, B 3, and B 4, kidneys, and adrenal glands.

Varicose veins: BP, especially BP 4, H 2B, rib cage to the side of the chest under the right armpit, directly onto the affected area.

Leukemia. BP, especially BP 2, spleen, B 3 and B 4 above spleen.

Liver. BP 1, back between the shoulder blades and below to the right.

Menstruation. For complications: BP 4, lower back, B 7, H 3.

Migraine. H 3, H 4, see in section on headaches, for women, abdomen, BP 4.

Mouth. Burned Tongue: On the mouth, under the tongue.

Stomatitis: BP, under the feet.

Mucus obstruction. For example, BP 3, stomach, bronchi, coughing, asthma, BP 5, pleura under the armpits.

Multiple sclerosis. BP, especially BP 3; H, especially H 2A, H 2B, H 3, H 4, especially motor nerves; B 1, B 1A, especially above the neck and between the shoulder blades, B 7, also affected areas, for example legs. With two practitioners: One person at the head, one at the feet.

Nausea. Morning Sickness: BP 1, BP 2, BP 3.

Motion Sickness: See section on **Balance**.

Neck. Ailment; BP, especially BP 3 and BP 4, H, especially H 3 and neck, B 1A, especially the neck/shoulder area and the 7th vertebrae.

Pain: Outer sides of the upper arms from elbow to shoulder.

Nervous breakdown. BP, especially BP 3, BP 4, and BP 5, H 2A, H 2B, H 3, H 4, from the side onto the head B 3, B 4, B 7.

Nosebleeds. H 3, H 5 to release tensions, BP 3, B 1A, B 2, shoulder blades.

Pain. In general: Over the area of pain, also B 3 and B 4.

For all bones in the body: B 1A, 7th vertebrae.

Hip or leg pains: Back, greater trochanter.

Pain in the arms: Back, tops of the shoulders, shoulder blades, shoulders and arms.

Arm, neck, and shoulder pains: Tops of the shoulders, collarbone at the shoulder, neck and shoulder.

Leg pains: Greater trochanter B 5–B 7, and directly onto the affected area.

Pleurisy. BP, especially BP 5, rib cage, under the armpits, H 1, apply light pressure under the eyebrows with your fingers, B 2 to–B 5.

Pneumonia. As described in pleurisy; rib cage, and back/lung, B 2–B 5, collarbone, and upper chest area.

Polyp (Nose). See description of sinus treatment, H 1, H 3.

Prostate. B 7; BP, especially BP 4; H 1, H 4.

Rheumatism. BP, B, B 3 and B 4, especially kidney.

Scars. On the scar.

Sciatica. B 5 and B 6, B 7, buttocks, back of the thighs, with your hands, make a connection between the heel of the foot and one of the buttocks, BP.

Scoliosis. BP and B over vertebrae.

Shock. Immediate treatment: BP 3, solar plexus and adrenal glands together or one at a time, then outer shoulders.

Later, after the shock: BP, especially BP 4, ovaries/prostate, B 3, B 4, especially kidneys and adrenal glands; H, H 3, H 4.

Sinus infection. BP, chest/bronchi, and collarbone, BP 5, H, H 1, slightly press finger onto bone under eyebrows and cheekbone, H 3, B 1, B 1A, neck/shoulder area.

Growth in the sinuses/polyps: see **Polyp.**

Skin. Red or brown spots on the skin: BP 1, liver (15–20 minutes).

Sleeplessness. BP 3, H, especially H 1, H 2B; B 1, B 1A, B 2, around the waist, collarbone area.

Spleen. BP 2, left side and back in the same area, B 3, B 4.

Sprains. Immediately: On the sprained area for 15–30 minutes.

After 24 hours: BP and onto the sprain, also greater trochanter, in case of leg or ankle injury.

Stings. Bee, mosquito, wasp: Treat the sting directly for 15–20 minutes.

Stomach. BP 2, BP 3, H 2B, and H 4, B 7.

Heartburn: H 3.

Digestive problems: BP 3, BP 4, BP 5, H 3, H 4, back B 3, and B 4, kidneys, and B 7, outside of upper arms.

Stroke. BP on the head, on the opposite side of the affected area of the body, for example, on the right side of the head if the left side of the body is affected.

Struma (Goiter). BP, especially BP 4, BP 5, B 7.

Surgery. A full treatment before and after the surgery.

Teething. On the baby's cheeks, the bottom of the feet.

Temper. Uncontrolled: BP 1, BP 2, liver, gallbladder, spleen, BP 3, BP 5, H 1, H 3.

Tension. BP, especially BP 3, BP 4, BP 5; H 1, H 3, H 4, on the side of the head.

Thyroid gland. In all cases where a treatment of the thyroid gland is necessary, also BP 4 and BP 7, while fasting and in cases of body fat/anorexia.

Tonsils. Infected: BP, H 1, H 3, H 5, B 3, B 4, kidneys.

Chronic: Treat regularly.

Toothache. On the painful area, H 1, H 2, upper and lower jaw.

Trauma. As described under "Shock," and the neck, B 1, B 1A, B 2–B 7.

Ulcer. Pylorus: BP 3, BP 4.

Duodenum: BP, especially below the waist, BP 3, H 1, slightly press nose bone where the cartilage starts.

Stomach: Outside of upper arms.

Weight problems. Body fat: Ovaries/prostate, BP 4 and thyroid gland, H 5.

Anorexia: Greater trochanter and side of the hips, then fat tissue.

24

REIKI SUPPORTS ALL OTHER FORMS OF THERAPY AND ALTERNATIVE METHODS OF HEALING

In general, it can be said that Reiki will automatically flow into any kind of hands-on treatment. With Reiki added, the treatment will be enriched and supported, for instance, in such therapies as: massage, foot reflexology, lymph drainage, soma massage, breathing therapy, rebalancing, shiatsu, rolfing, acupressure, acupuncture, or cosmetic massages.

Reiki is especially useful for all those in healing professions because they will be charged, along with their patients, with every treatment.

Other methods of healing that respond positively to Reiki are: rebirthing, autogenic training (AT), yoga, meditation, Bach flower remedies and California flower essences, homeopathy, Verana color foils, prescribed detox and fasting treatments, psychotherapy, music therapy, crystals, and precious stones.

The Verana Color-Foil System

The Verana Color-Foil system harmonizes wonderfully with Reiki, and there have been very good related experiences. This system helps the bioenergetics transformation of body, mind, and soul. It was developed by Vera A. Suchanek and is based on twenty years of research and observing cosmic energies and their influences on humans, animals, and plants. The color foils enable the intake of the vertical rays from the sun to the earth and vice versa. They assist in connecting with the horizontal waves for the transmission and reception of information, in order to be able to live in physical and spiritual harmony with the cosmos and nature.

Vera Suchanek says: "We live today in a time of major changes in the energies of the earth and the cosmos. Because we are a part of nature, we have no other choice but to go with the flow of these changes in order to survive. For one year, I conducted regular radiesthetic checkups on the energetic changes every two hours. Later, I developed a sensitivity which enabled me to immediately recognize any change. The changes in the atmosphere did not appear with regularity."

There are many different color foils with different effects, for example in cases of cancer, multiple sclerosis, or AIDS, and so forth. The foils are also individually and intuitively chosen and measured. They are made by hand, and their use is very simple. You look through the foils for one to two minutes, or carry them, and the body responds to them intuitively.

25

KIRLIAN PHOTOGRAPHY AND REIKI

After many years of research, and with the help of their high-frequency photography, the two Russian scientists Semjon and Walentina Kirlian succeeded in making the micro-structural, bioenergetics radiation (aura) of the human body, leaves, or other objects,visible to the human eye.

Today, Kirlian photography is used by many doctors and healers for energetic analysis (see Peter Mandel, Energy Emission Analysis) as a way to see bioenergetics disturbances early on. These disturbances include fatigue, illness, and changing moods in the energy body of the human being —an illness exists in the energy body long before it is physically apparent.

The Kirlian photographs shown here were made available by a Reiki practitioner. They show the bioenergetics field of a hand before and after a mental Reiki treatment (2nd Degree), which was carried out on the head for only a few seconds:

"The pictures shown were taken on August 2, 1989 at about 9 PM. I took pictures over the course of several months, always before and after Reiki treatments. Most striking were the experiments I made with mental treatments of the 2nd Degree. The pictures were made within five minutes, as we had a color laboratory. Immediately after the first picture, I gave this person—a man—a short mental treatment (light and love) as he was standing up. The changes that took place in the second Kirlian photography can hardly be put into words. I repeated these experiments with the mental treatment several times, and each time I felt deep respect and gratitude for this wonderful power, especially for the enormous energy of thought."

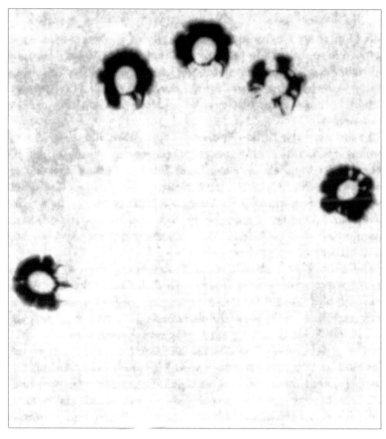

First picture, before the mental Reiki treatment (S 8–2 Ho20889)

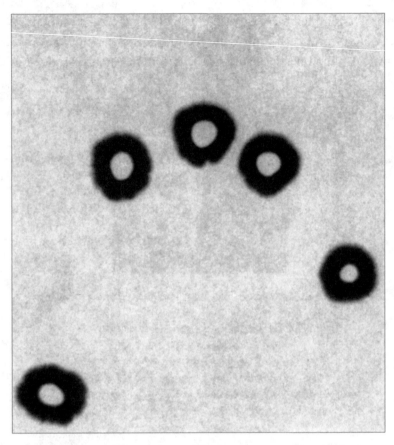

Second picture, after the mental Reiki treatment (S 8–2 Ho
020889). The stronger energetic radiation is clearly visible.

A PRAYER OF ST. FRANCIS OF ASSISI

"Lord, make me an instrument of Your Peace.
Where there is hatred, let me sow love,
Where there is injury, pardon,
Where there is doubt, faith,
Where there is despair, hope,
Where there is darkness, light,
And where there is sadness, joy.

O Divine Master, grant that I may.
Not so much seek to be consoled,
   as to console;
To be understood, as to understand;
To be loved, as to love;
For it is in giving that we receive—
It is in pardoning that we are pardoned,
And it is in dying that we are born to
   eternal life.

26

My Path with Reiki

Brigitte Müller, Reiki Master/Teacher

I found my life's purpose in Reiki. I had said the prayer of the holy St. Francis of Assisi long before I was led to Reiki, and my prayers were heard. While traveling in the United States in January 1981, I met the Reiki Master Mary McFadyen in Northern California. She just *happened* to pick me up from the airport. As we were driving in her car she told me about Reiki. I was listening with great interest. When I asked her whether I could have a Reiki treatment, she told me it was even possible to transmit Reiki in such a way that I could have the healing power in my own hands. I immediately asked Mary if there was a workshop anytime soon. She told me none was planned, but she could initiate me alone, without a workshop. The next day she agreed to it.

I was staying in a small cabin in a forest near Nevada City. Deer were walking outside my window and I was far away from the busy everyday life of the world. It was a perfect place to receive my initiation into the 1st Degree Reiki. Mary explained the treatment, and we practiced on each other. Those were wonderful days, and I am so grateful to Mary for bringing Reiki to me at that time. In the beginning I could hardly grasp that I now had *healing hands*, but I felt a lot of power and warmth in my hands and applied them tentatively on myself to try Reiki. At the same time, I had a burning desire to give someone else Reiki, but this had to wait for a while.

First I flew back to Los Angeles. There I rented a room from an eighty-year-old lady, and a few days later, I had an opportunity to successfully use Reiki when, all of a sudden, I heard yelling from the kitchen. The elderly lady had put her fingers into the garbage disposal to free a piece of orange peel that was stuck, but she had forgotten to turn off the switch, and her fingertips had been cut by the blades. She was bleeding profusely, and I immediately put on a pressure-bandage and also pressed my hands onto the wound. To my surprise, the bleeding stopped very quickly—it was just like the moment when Dr. Usui treated his injured foot with Reiki to stop the bleeding. We drove to the hospital because the wounds needed stitches. Upon arrival I applied my hands again, and the lady calmed down quickly. A nurse instructed me to leave the room, much to the dismay of the old lady. She insisted that I stay with her because my hands "felt so good." This was my first Reiki treatment. Every day I treated her hand which, to the surprise of the doctors, healed very quickly.

A short while later I flew back to Germany where my parents received my first Reiki treatments. After a few self-healing reactions, they felt very charged. My bulldog Etzel also liked Reiki a lot. He would lie down comfortably, sigh, then snore when I put my hands on him. My mother wanted to learn Reiki right away, and some of my friends also wanted to receive the initiation after I had familiarized them with Reiki. In 1981, I organized the first-ever Reiki workshop in Germany (Hamburg) with Mary McFadyen, then held a second one in Frankfurt. I translated the workshop's lectures into German, which gave me an opportunity to gain workshop experience. After my 1st Degree initiation in the U.S., I immediately felt it was my calling to be a Reiki Master. I received the 2nd Degree Reiki during Mary's stay in Germany. At this time, I was also training to become a naturopath.

After passing the naturopath exam, I contacted Phyllis Lei Furumoto, Mrs. Hawayo Takata's granddaughter, to ask about the Reiki Master initiation. I flew to the United States and Canada in

January of 1983, and traveled with Phyllis for several weeks. She closely examined my abilities as we drove through the beautiful Canadian countryside. I met several Reiki Masters, and everywhere we went, I was taken in as family. We participated in some Reiki workshops, gave Reiki treatments, and eventually our journey took us to Phyllis's house in Canada. After three weeks there, she informed me that she would initiate me as a Reiki Master/Teacher. I was overjoyed!

The time for my initiation came on January 27, 1983. It took place in a small wooden cabin that belonged to another Reiki Master and Mary McFadyen was present. We had waded through the snow to get to it, and once inside, the first thing we did was make a small fire.

The initiation itself was a very deep experience for me and I was very happy. That afternoon, Phyllis began a 1st Degree workshop, and for the first time I was allowed to give an initiation. I felt a great inner peace and much gratitude that I was allowed to be an instrument for this divine power. My hands were tingling and vibrating, and I felt a pulsating energy throughout my entire body.

Phyllis had some wonderful plums in her freezer, and I baked a German plum cake with whipped cream for the occasion. As we celebrated the day with our Reiki students, I thanked God from deep within my heart for his blessing and his grace. We were all abundantly cared for on this day of my Master initiation.

During the days that followed, I received further training, and we also had a 2nd Degree workshop. In the course of those weeks, Phyllis and I found a deep inner connection with each other. It was a very intense time, and I felt the need for a peaceful retreat to let the Master energy settle. We parted, and I went to Southern California to the Self–Realization Fellowship in Encinitas. This community was founded by Paramahansa Yogananda, author of *Autobiography of a Yogi*, which he wrote there. This was the ideal place to retreat. I spent wonderful days meditating and praying. The meditation garden with its beautiful flowers, whispering streams and a pond with giant goldfish, directly on a cliff over the Pacific was refreshment for my soul. This was where I was able to prepare myself for the life of a Reiki Master. I could clearly feel the blessing and vibrations of the enlightened Master Paramahansa Yogananda, and I was very grateful to be there.

After those days of inner searching I was ready to return to Germany and begin to undertake my life's work. Since I was the first Reiki Master/Teacher in Germany and only a few people knew about Reiki, I was really a pioneer and there was a lot to do. Workshops had to be organized, and the necessary tasks were accomplished with help from the many who supported me then and are still helping me now—to them all I owe a great debt of gratitude.

A new part of my life had begun, and this new work filled me entirely. It is such a beautiful feeling to be connected with everyone in a workshop group, to grow together, and become unified through love = Reiki.

My Personal Perceptions of Reiki

During my years of being a Reiki Master/Teacher, and through meeting all the people participating in my workshops, I have come to feel Reiki in my heart and soul, but I would like to convey in words how I personally perceive Reiki.

I have had deep inner perceptions and experiences, especially during Reiki initiations, because the Reiki initiation touches our innermost being. This inner being is the divine spark or the divine Self within us, our immortal essence. It is like a reunification with God's Presence in our hearts, reconnecting us with our center of love. Our innermost essence is love, and it is always present. We are love. However, many have forgotten this. Now the beam of love flows through the entire being, and a jubilant joy fills us. The inner source, which may have been blocked, once again begins to bubble. Our heart is connected with our hands. The hands bless everything and everybody with love. Love is the strongest force in the universe. It is the binding force that keeps planets, stars, suns, and our Earth on track. We can feel that we are a part of creation, and also that everything exists within ourselves, just like a drop of the ocean contains the whole ocean.

Through the gentle touch of our hands we transmit Reiki, which is love = light = Universal Life Energy. This brings us close to ourselves—we are once again touching ourselves. Our entire being is filled with it, and the light glows from our eyes, heart, hands, and bodies. Because love has the highest frequency, we experience a transformation into this higher frequency. Love is light! We are light! When all of a sudden it gets brighter in us, our dark sides will also be revealed. Love = light = Reiki also shines light on the things within ourselves that we don't like to see very much and enables us to accept them with equal love. Being able to see or recognize yourself is the beginning of the change. We now have a key in our hands that lets us form our lives the way we like. Reiki helps us find our blocks and obstacles. Because we apply our Reiki hands on our own bodies every day and let in more and more light, we become more loving, harmonious, balanced, and understanding with ourselves and others. We begin to accept and love ourselves the way we are.

For me a time of inner growth had begun. I learned a lot from my students in the workshops, because we are all teacher and student at the same time. We teach what we learn ourselves, and everyone learns from everyone. It was a joy to see how hearts opened and unified everyone in love at the end of the workshop. We are always connected with this vibration because love has no limits.

Reiki took me to many countries where I had been invited to give workshops. I had the distinct wish to bring Reiki to the Eastern European countries. Before I was initiated as a Reiki Master, Phyllis Lei Furumoto had asked me, "Why do you want to become a Reiki Master?" I told her I wanted to bring the Reiki light and healing power to Germany as a way to contribute to the unification of the German people, and all other people; to heal the wounds of the war.

I had lived in the former East Germany as a child, and, because of this, my 1988 trip to Poland was an experience I will never forget. As I arrived, the "Week of Healing and Holistic Being" was taking place in Krakow, and it was the first official event of its kind in Poland. It featured lectures, discussions, free seminars, and meditation workshops. Teachers from around the world had traveled to Krakow to take part in the event. The Reiki workshops were so popular that we could hardly keep up with the work. In only four days, 270 people were initiated into the 1st Degree, which was a real transformation for me. During this time I had great support from some Reiki friends who had traveled with me from Germany. People were searching for peace and light so strongly that it was a great pleasure to see their change and their glowing faces in the course of the workshops. Since that time, I have trained and initiated a Reiki Master in Poland, so that Reiki can spread further there.

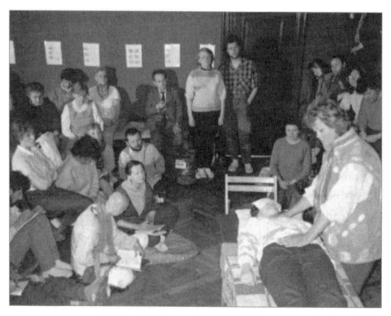

Brigitte Müller during a Reiki Workshop in Poland

Then, the Berlin Wall opened up here in Germany, and that was a joyful day in my life.

Reiki led me to further self-discovery. Toward the end of 1983, I participated in a workshop with Elizabeth Kübler-Ross. This was very moving and I learned to take responsibility for my own emotions and experiences. I especially learned to be aware of unfinished business coming to the surface, and being conscious of people pushing my buttons, or me pushing theirs, as often happens in workshops. I realized that the clearer I became with myself, the better I was able to help the people in my workshops.

During a stay in the U.S., I bought the book *Loving Relationships* by Sondra Ray. Reading this book and working with its exercises, I immediately saw my own *patterns,* and knew I wanted to take part in the Loving Relationship Training as soon as possible. This training is about realizing the partially unconscious behavior patterns connected to the trauma of birth and childhood, and transforming them into self-love and joyful, loving relationships. I participated in the training twice in 1986, May in Stockholm and November in London, and they were both revealing and healing for me. In years to come, I repeatedly participated in ten-day follow-up trainings in Hawaii, the Bahamas, and Spain. In addition to the group rebirthing sessions, I received personal, one-on-one sessions, and found that Reiki was very supportive in this rebirthing process where a lot of things were released and integrated within me. These workshops helped me accept and love myself and have come to mean a great deal to me. I became more aware and began to watch my thoughts, because thoughts are creative, they manifest themselves. We ourselves create our own circumstances through our thoughts; we can, in effect, choose ourselves.

This also corresponds with the spiritual rules of life. I remember the beggars in the history of Reiki who didn't want to change their thoughts and perceptions of life. In the past, I always looked for love, acknowledgment, and peace on the outside, and now I am realizing that the source of all this is within myself: the source of divine love. The moment we are able to find love within ourselves, we become the masters of our lives; it isn't until then that we can really love. We become free, we become love in action and we won't need anything from the outside any longer because everything we send out will return to us. This love will return to us many times over, eventually reuniting with the source, so the cycle closes itself.

In my years of intense work, I have had countless experiences with the Reiki healing force. At times there have even been spontaneous healings after only one or two treatments. My hands have always been ready for immediate use, even in emergencies and accidents. On several occasions I have been able to calm people after accidents, and relieve their pain and shock.

A Selection of Shared Experiences

Reiki Helps to Avoid Operation

The eighty-three-year-old husband of a friend got an infection and experienced a painful enlargement of the testicles after a urethra examination. My friend, who is a 2nd Degree Reiki practitioner, immediately began a treatment directly onto the testicles (if direct contact is not appropriate in your situation, give Reiki within a few inches of distance). Twice a week, I helped with the treatment. The doctors at the hospital decided that one of the testicles should be surgically removed, but postponed the operation because of bacteria in the urine, during which time we kept giving intensive Reiki treatments. After four or five weeks, the size of the testicle was reduced, and within four months it was back to normal, making surgery unnecessary.

Reiki for A Dog's Life

When my male dog boxer, Etzel, was about the age of five, he developed a heart defect and the veterinarian prescribed an allopathic heart medication, which I gave him every day for many years. After my initiation into 1st Degree Reiki, I gave him a lot of treatments, and we were able to slowly reduce the dosage of the medication. At a later examination by the veterinarian, no heart irregularities were detected, and the medication was stopped entirely. But when he was nearly twelve, Etzel became ill with leukemia. Again, he received many treatments from me and afterward, he always jumped up and licked my hands in joy. At times he got very weak, especially while taking walks. He would simply sit down and not walk again until I put my hands around him. Soon after that, he would be charged again, stand up, and jump around. If I removed my hands before he had received enough, though, he would simply keep sitting. During his last hour, I stayed with him, giving Reiki, and his soul was able to peacefully move into another dimension. After his heart stopped beating, I held him in my arms for an hour and he looked as if he was asleep in peace. Reiki helped me stay calm during this difficult time. When my Mother touched my liver during a Reiki treatment the following day, I was able to freely let my tears flow. A few months later, I finished the grieving process—acceptance and integration of pain—in a workshop with Dr. Elizabeth Kuebler-Ross. Thank you, Elizabeth, from the depths of my heart.

Reiki Healing High on a Mountain

During a morning Reiki workshop, a lady in another workshop at the hotel injured her foot, landing on it in a bad way while dancing, which resulted in a stretched ligament—within seconds, two swellings the size of eggs had formed on the outside of her ankle. She was brought into our Reiki room with ice packs on her foot. Four or five of us immediately began giving Reiki for several hours—head, front of the body, kidneys/adrenal glands, and directly onto the foot. I started out giving Reiki with the ice pack on the foot, and later I alternately treated with and without the ice. Emotions were heightened, and the lady cried. We had also called a doctor to see whether the foot was broken. However, because we were on a 3500 foot mountain, the doctor—from the army—did not come until the evening. Meanwhile, the lady's foot had become even more swollen and was turning blue and green. To us, it appeared to be going through an accelerated healing process. When the doctor arrived, he confirmed that her foot was not broken, but said it would take about two weeks for her to be able to put any weight on the foot. He left her some pain pills, but it turned out she didn't have to take them because Reiki was easing her pain. Even at night she did not have any pain. The next morning, we continued the Reiki group treatment on her for about two hours. By the afternoon, the swelling had receded and all that was left was a small bruise around the ankle. By 6 PM, the lady was able to stand up without crutches, put weight on her foot, and *walk*. And it had only been thirty hours since the accident—that is how much Reiki accelerated the healing process.

Alcohol-Fueled Seizure Stopped with Reiki

During a workshop in Stuttgart, I was walking back to the meeting room after lunch with a participant when we saw a young man lying hunched up and motionless on the sidewalk. With him was a large black dog on a leash. People were standing around him saying, "There is nothing we can do, it is much too late." We approached the man, got on our knees, and began giving him Reiki. The participant put her hands on his kidneys, and without touching him, I put mine around his head. He smelled like alcohol and was not responding to my words. The dog stayed completely calm and looked at us. After a while, I put my hands directly on his head. After a few minutes, he regained consciousness, but when I tried to remove my hands, he said, "Please leave them where they are, they feel so good." We asked if he was diabetic, but he wasn't. It turned out he was epileptic and drinking a beer had triggered a seizure. We continued the treatment, and after a while he began to sob, snuggling in my lap like a child seeking protection. After about ten minutes, he calmed down, got up off the sidewalk, and was clear again, at which time we asked for his address so his wife could be contacted. Meanwhile the police had been called, and by the time they arrived, he was feeling completely fine. When we said goodbye, he thanked us very much and told us he was about to start an alcohol detox program. Once again the divine force was able to help.

I felt deep within myself that the time had come for the next important step on my Master's path, and felt ready when Phyllis Lei Furumoto gave me the blessing and empowerment to undertake the training and initiation of Reiki Masters/Teachers. At the end of 1988, I initiated the first Reiki Master/Teacher in Poland; many more followed, and more are currently in training.

Being initiated as a Master does not mean you have learned everything there is to learn. On the contrary, it is an admission into the *higher school of life*. For me, it means being ready for change, and revitalizing old ways of thinking to receive everything with love and gratitude, flow with the energy, transform energies, be one with God's presence in my heart, and surrender to this guidance within.

Reiki has transformed my entire quality of life, even my life itself. Reiki is a miracle that shows me new miracles every day. My deepest wish is that many more people in the world could receive Reiki initiation, so that everyone could come closer and become a large family living in peace, love, and harmony on this earth. We are all One in spirit and in love.

I am grateful for God's grace, for the blessings I experience in my life, and for being allowed to be an *instrument*.

27

My Path with Reiki

Horst H. Günther, Reiki Master/Teacher

With gratitude and complete trust in the creativity of the universe, I want to begin with excerpts from the writings of the great physicist Max Planck:

"As a physicist, a man who has served in the sober sciences and the description of matter for my entire life, I am free of the suspicion of being seen as a dreamer. With this in mind, I say the following as a result of my research of the atom: no matter exists by itself. All matter is created and exists only through the force that causes the vibration of the parts of the atom and that holds it together into the smallest solar system of an atom. Behind this force, we have to assume a conscious and intelligent spirit. This spirit is the origin of all matter. It is not the visible, transient matter that is actual, true, and real, because matter would not exist without spirit by itself. It is the invisible, immortal spirit that is real. But since the spirit cannot exist by itself, and since every spirit is part of a being, we must accept the existence of spiritual beings. But even spiritual beings cannot create themselves and must have been created. I do not hesitate to give this mysterious creator the same name that most cultures on earth have given it for thousands of years: God!"

* * *

As a young man, I started working in business and climbed the career ladder through various positions in the German business system. I reached a point where I began to realize that climbing up was not really going anywhere and I had to admit to myself, and especially to my family, that my life was solely dedicated to the company I worked for. I was faced with the questions of awakening: Is this all? Family or career? Are there other ways? Who can help me? How can I help myself?

Looking back, I can understand how, at that point, I began the path of self-mastery. Through several years of self-discovery, I continued in business, but also learned rebirthing and trained in white-water kayaking—both were very important on this path. I was often confronted with situations in which I had to overcome fear and was forced to move into completely new and unknown areas of myself. I thank my teachers and friends, Dr. Wolfgang Strasser and Bertold Wichmann, for their special association with me. I practiced the rebirthing technique I had been taught for almost five years by an accomplished psychologist, and I thank Angela Rudhardt for our intensive practice.

I still felt, however, that I had to keep growing. Then one day I saw a flyer for a workshop that said, "Reiki—Heal Yourself! given by Brigitte Müller." It sounded so interesting that I convinced my wife, Edith, to go with me to the workshop. This decision in the beginning of 1984 opened a new life for us—we just didn't know it yet.

During this 1st Degree workshop, I was surprised to realize that something was changing within me, and especially in my hands: My wife and I had received the gift of healing hands and we were so inspired by this new sensation that, immediately after the workshop, we began to give each other treatments several times a week. The desire to learn more about Reiki grew in us, and we told Brigitte that we wanted to receive the 2nd Degree Reiki, which we did, later that same year. While broadening our insights about understanding it in general, we began to study the specific meaning of the Oku Den, the deeper wisdom of Reiki. The most eventful times came after each workshop, when we began to integrate what we had learned into our daily lives. We could hardly believe what we were able to do with Reiki, and became so Reiki-ized that we began to enthusiastically organize workshops for Brigitte. During this time, I came to the clear realization of how phenomenal it was to experience the positive changes in people during a weekend workshop, and how wonderful it felt to be allowed to experience this.

One day Brigitte put into words what I had unconsciously felt: that she could imagine me becoming a Reiki Master. I played with this thought for several months and often talked about it with my wife until it suddenly became clear to me that I wanted to become a Reiki Master/Teacher. My next step was to write Phyllis Lei Furumoto, the Grand Master of the Usui System, and apply for the training and initiation to be a Reiki Master. She replied with an invitation to a self-assessment workshop in the United States. To me this was a sign that I was on the right path so I traveled from Frankfurt, Germany to Boise, Idaho.

There were five of us future Reiki Masters participating in the workshop. We approached each other very openly, and everyone had a chance to share and work on things within themselves. During the course of the workshop, we became mirrors for each other, in order to see ourselves more clearly. It was left open how many participants Phyllis would initiate into Reiki Masters. Then, on the last night—it was already moving towards morning—Phyllis said, "At sunrise I will initiate Horst as a Reiki Master."

Since I had not counted on being initiated, it came as a complete surprise, and a very moving experience to be initiated as a Reiki Master at sunrise on July 6th, 1985 in the mountains of Bogus Basin, Idaho. Phyllis Lei Furumoto, Michael Hartly, Paul and Susan Mitchell, Brigitte Müller, Hiltrud Marg, and I, climbed a beautiful mountain at 6:30 AM and were treated to a wonderful panoramic view of the surrounding mountains, forests, and desert. We could all feel the exceptional energies that were released when Phyllis said, "Now is the right time." There are no words to describe how much

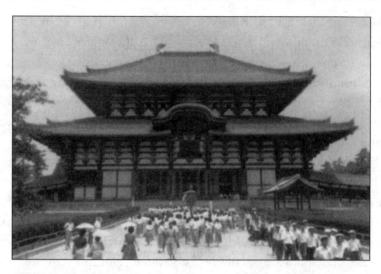

Temple Nara Daibutsu. In 1987, my Reiki path also brought me to the important Reiki cities of Japan, Kyoto and Tokyo, as well as to Japan's holy mountain, Fujiyama. My family and I had many uplifting moments while traveling through this beautiful country with Reiki as our constant companion. We kept thinking how it was here that Dr. Usui rediscovered and unfolded Reiki. In Nara, the old city of the emperor, close to Kyoto, I took the above picture of Japan's largest temple, the Nara Daibutsu.

deep gratitude I feel towards Phyllis for transferring this energy to me through the initiation.

I stayed in Boise for the Master training with Phyllis, and Susan and Paul Mitchell, who gave me the opportunity to assist him in one of his Reiki workshops. Before returning to Germany, I went to visit the Yogananda ashram in Encinitas, California to quietly retreat and reflect on the work of the past weeks. All through this time I received great support from my wife, Edith, and our Reiki Master friend Brigitte Müller. And I still think of all the great friends who helped me with their trust and practical support as I began my practice, and who continue to do so today.

During the entire trip—the long flights and waiting periods, especially—I was self-treating my right elbow with Reiki. Several years before, I had been diagnosed with tennis elbow and had received medications and injections for it, but the symptoms kept returning. Although I cannot say exactly how many hours I treated my elbow in the course of the trip, one thing is certain: by the time I arrived back in Germany, I no longer felt any pain and could move my arm as if nothing had ever happened to it. To this day, thank God, I have had no further symptoms of tennis elbow.

At home, days, weeks, and months were filled with the tasks of my work and Reiki. At that time, *The Blue Reiki Book* was translated and printed in German, and Brigitte and I also wrote *The White Reiki Guidebook*, which we distributed to our workshop participants. A lot of Reiki workshops were taking place, and we held the first international Reiki Master conference in Friedrichsdorf, Taunus, Germany. It was all a wonderful time, full of rich experiences, but I was still working as a businessman, and felt a deep urge to stop working and give myself to Reiki completely.

How I was to do this became clear on October 27, 1986. Early in the morning of that day, something extraordinary happened, which led to a complete change in my life. For reasons I can't explain, I fell sideways in front of a moving car, and for reasons just as inexplicable, I somehow turned myself, or maybe I *was* turned, in such a way that I landed lying lengthwise between the two front wheels of the car. The driver was able to stop the car just as my head lay under the car's front grill. Although I had many internal and external injuries, I was completely conscious during the entire event, and was intensely aware of the pain and everything going on around me. I felt clearly, "Now everything is over." I later realized the depth of the message, that every end brings a new beginning.

I was forced to rest in order to heal. I was also about to change my life, giving up my then current occupation and dedicating myself to what I was called for. While recovering, I had to be my own patient, giving myself Reiki as best I could, and working with the

2nd Degree Reiki. My loving wife Edith also gave me Reiki every day, and friends, such as Dagmar Bock, helped as well during the difficult first few days. And in addition to the many distant Reiki treatments I received, Phyllis, Brigitte, and other Reiki friends, came to treat me directly. I will never forget how much my Austrian Reiki friends helped me over the telephone. It was a tidal wave of willingness to help that I had never before experienced. A spontaneous healing network had formed itself and made me feel deeply thankful. With all this support, I began planning my future while still in the hospital, and was able to go home in about two weeks.

Although it took two more years of exhausting difficulties, it was a joy to succeed in the practical realization of my independence, and receive the gift of my own life.

A Few Significant Shared Experiences

A Mother's Help from Reiki

An acquaintance called one night and asked me to drive to a hospital in faraway Rheinland-Pfalz to help Julia, a forty-one-year-old mother of two children who had advanced cancer. She had been told she would never get out of her bed again because her bones would break like glass due to her bone-marrow cancer. Julia was physically, spiritually, and mentally in very bad shape, so I began working with her on a mental level, and gave her Reiki at the same time. I visited her often, and we had long conversations over the phone. At a certain point I initiated her into the 1st Degree Reiki, so she could treat herself in my absence. About six weeks later, she left the hospital in an ambulance, but responsible for herself. Her general condition was greatly improved, and she was able to live with her severe illness.

At home, Julia was treated by her family doctor, a sister who cared for her on a daily basis, and a doctor friend who worked with her on a spiritual level from time to time. I visited her often, and it was always an extraordinary gift to be able to treat this woman with

Reiki. One day on the phone, she said, "You won't have to come to my place next time we meet. I'm driving again and will meet you halfway. I'll take you out to dinner." I felt overwhelmed with surprise and gratitude, and was, as well, deeply respectful of the universe. She did drive herself to the agreed-upon place, and as we embraced each other, tears of joy and thankfulness flowed from us both. Once more, I felt grateful to have been allowed such an experience in my life.

Julia ultimately moved into her parent's house where she had loving people by her side. This helped her understand that there are universal, divine rules which become reality, though they are often incomprehensible to us. During her last days on earth, she kept reassuring us that the last two years had been the most intensive and meaningful time of her life. Understanding this, Julia was able to let go, and left us in peace and harmony.

Reiki for a Dog's Life

Reiki works on animals beyond the physical level, as in the case of our dog Anka, a female Dalmatian.

Anka had been with us for twelve adventure-filled years and had become a real member of the family. But as she got older, she began to have physical difficulties, especially in the hip. During our walks, Anka had to stop often and would sometimes lie down. When we gave her Reiki, she would resume walking at a quick pace with no visible difficulties, but it became clear to us that she was reaching the end of her days. The intervals between treatments became shorter and shorter, and then we had to give her Reiki every day. One day she was doing very badly, and it seemed as if nothing helped anymore. I still remember it clearly: Anka stood in our kitchen and was not able to move at all. I looked at her, put my hands on her head and body, and the look in her eyes as she gazed at me was intensely powerful. There are types of vibrations expressed through the physical organs—in this case the dog's eyes—that you can only try to describe. The message I received in her eyes was that she completely understood what was happening, simultaneously accepting it as a release. There were no signs of fight or discomfort in her, although she must have been in a lot of pain. And unforgettable for me was the great thankfulness that her eyes were expressing, like a wave of unconditional love. As Anka lay dying that day, we accompanied her transformation with distant Reiki. It was important for us to send her on her way with light and love.

Reiki's Help in a Diving Emergency

I want to encourage all Reiki practitioners to be prepared with their healing hands when emergencies occur. My wife, son Armin, and I were in Turkey for a few days and Armin was enjoying his hobby of skin diving. One day we watched from the shore as he went out in a small boat with another boy and their diving instructor. Everything seemed to be fine, but all of a sudden we saw a person surface in the water, helping another person in the water. The distance was too far for us to see who it was, but we could see clearly that one of the divers was receiving first aid out there in the water. We immediately began sending out distant Reiki. One diver, we didn't know which, was pulled into the small boat and my wife and I were obviously very worried, since one of divers was our son. As the boat came closer to the shore, we could see that the diving instructor was steering the boat and our son had his hands on the chest of the other diver, who appeared motionless. Suddenly there were several women next to us, and one, the boy's mother, began to weep loudly. Everyone helped to get the boat and its passengers onto the shore. Without hesitating, I asked the boy's mother if I could treat him until a doctor arrived. She looked at me skeptically when I explained that I would apply my hands, but after considering the situation, she agreed to my therapy. I began using the emergency Reiki positions and started to communicate with the boy's higher self. After about fifteen minutes, he opened his eyes and looked helplessly and weakly at the crowd around him as it dawned on him that he was being treated. His mother was beside herself with joy and thanked me, but the boy did not want to be touched any more. I recommended that they consult a doctor immediately. After the excitement settled down, our son told us that the boy, who was about his age, had begun to panic underwater and had resurfaced much too fast without his mask. During that moment of shock and fear, my son Armin had already begun an emergency Reiki treatment in the water.

Emergency Help in a Parasailing Incident

Another time I was in the South of France with my family. One of the attractions offered on the beach was parasailing. We went to look because I had always wanted to try it, and I ended up having a wonderful flight. After I landed, I watched a young woman prepare for her turn in the air. She was running fast, trying to get off the ground, but was unable to steer her parachute quite right and some wind came along and hit her from the side, and she ended up being uncontrollably dragged over the beach and the shore. The wayward parachute ripped a wooden fence out of the ground and hit another woman in the head. That woman fell to the ground, crying out loudly while blood was running down her head. As everyone stared helplessly at her, an inner flash went through me and I ran to the scene, yelling for someone to call a doctor, and at the same time beginning emergency treatment, which also works for shock and fear. Despite her open head wound, the woman stopped screaming and was able to consciously look at me. What I saw in her eyes was that she felt taken care of and had quiet trust in me for the ten minutes I worked with her until the paramedics arrived.

Reiki's Help in Letting Go

I had an especially deep experience with my friend George's father during his last hours. He was in the hospital, fighting for his life on earth. He did not want to let go, and he expressed this by sitting up in bed, rocking up and down, and trying to literally hold on to what could not be held anymore. That was how I found him. Everything had been done for him; he was well taken care of, medically and technically. In the presence of his family, I put my hands on him in various specific places and after three or four minutes, I felt his tightness and cramps loosen. He stopped rocking back and forth, which surprised everyone, since I hadn't said a word to him. I did, however, have constant eye contact with him and was able to read the sudden change in his eyes. Although unable to speak, I could read his eyes saying, "I have understood, everything is all right, I am now able to let go." And he did. For me, this was a completely new experience, and it took me some time to integrate it and come to understand it as a gift.

Reiki's Effect on My Everyday Life

On this path, I am surprised at the way Reiki affects things connected with my everyday life—often in relation to objects or technical machinery. Here is just one example of that.

On a break during the Reiki Master conference on the big island of Hawaii, a lady from our camp, a fellow Reiki Master from Greece, and I were driven to the next, larger town. Along the way, we had to stop for gas. There were two keys, one for the ignition and one for the gas cap. When the gas-station attendant returned the keys to the driver, he mixed them up, and suddenly the gas-cap key was stuck in the ignition, and nothing would move it. It wouldn't come out or turn either way. The driver, the attendant, the Greek lady, and I all gave it a try, each with our own little tricks and ways, but nothing happened. Sitting in the back seat, I sent Reiki to the key, but there was no movement. The gas attendant then called someone else, who came over with a huge monkey wrench such as I had never seen before. Our driver took one look at it and asked this person to please stop, it wasn't even her car; she had only borrowed it from someone else in the camp. So, before this guy with his huge wrench could do any damage I asked to give Reiki one more try. I traded seats with the driver, and began to give the ignition Reiki. After about three or four minutes, feeling it was done, I took my hands away, touched the key with my thumb and index finger, pulled

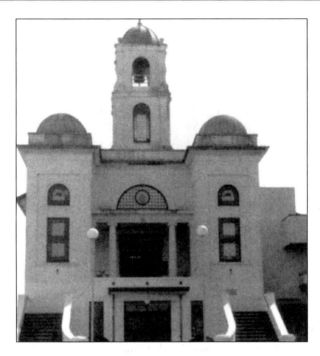

Mrs. Hawayo Takata's Resting Place. On our way home from the church to where we were staying in Kalani Honua, we received an extra special goodbye gift from the heavens—a beam of light from above—which I was able to capture in the following photo:

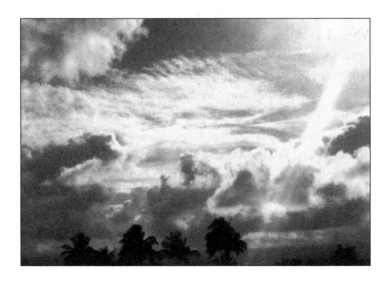

up lightly, and without any force the key came loose. Besides my Greek colleague and I, nobody around understood what had just happened, but I was very grateful for Reiki. Not so for the attendant with the huge wrench—he actually looked quite disappointed, as if we had gotten in the way of his special service.

In the course of the conference, we also visited Mrs. Hawayo Takata's last resting place in Hilo, Hawaii. The photo on the previous page shows the church where Mrs. Takata's urn is kept.

I believe that Reiki has allowed my creative abilities to unfold. Because of the integration of its power into my daily life, I have been able to recognize the needs of the people around me, and have discovered ways to meet them. Out of this came a method of life-supporting treatments, which my wife and I have been teaching in workshops since 1989, and which we call CREAMO.

In Helen J. Haberly's book, *Reiki: Hawayo Takata's Story*, I found a parallel connection when I read about a student of Mrs. Takata's who had developed her creativity through Reiki. In its own way, this wonderful power helps to find and unfold a person's talent.

I want to encourage all people, in whatever kinds of careers or occupations they have, to learn and use Reiki; to give it to our families, neighbors, friends, animals, and plants. This is what our planet needs so desperately, a special kind of healing: Love.

When I look back today, I realize how Reiki has completely changed my life. Being a Reiki Master, I am aware that I can still contribute to the spreading of Reiki, so its loving energy will find its way to all people. My own personal development reached a completely new dimension when Phyllis Lei Furumoto gave me permission to train and initiate other Reiki Masters and I feel a humble gratitude for being allowed to carry Reiki on in this way. Besides the U.S. and Europe, it is being taught in India, Brazil, Africa, Hungary, and Russia—all over the world.

My wife Edith and I are very grateful to transmit light and love to all living things with Reiki.

AFTERWORD

We hope you have enjoyed this book on Reiki, and we would like to thank you for taking the time to give yourself an inside view of the Reiki healing methods.

If you now feel the desire to receive *the gift of healing hands*, we hope that your path will lead you to *your* Reiki Master.

If you have already been initiated into Reiki, we are glad to have connected with you, and hope this book has given you further inspiration.

May love, peace, and joy be with you!

—Brigitte Müller and Horst H. Günther

IMPORTANT NOTE

Again and again, we get letters or calls from people who went to a Reiki seminar and did not experience any change of energy in their hands, or did not benefit from any healing process—just the opposite. These people sometimes complained they felt worse and did not experience anything our book describes.

When some of these people finally had the chance to be initiated by us into the 1st and 2nd degree, they affirmed the presence of Reiki in themselves, and said the healing process *did* occur. Because an experienced Reiki Master/Teacher is crucial to the process of effectively receiving the Reiki initiations and healing, we want to raise your awareness of what to look for in choosing suitably and well.

In recent years, many people have participated in Reiki crash courses that do not adhere to the traditional method of learning Reiki, and this has diluted and abused the practice of Reiki. People who became so-called Reiki Masters this way did not generally develop their capacity to transfer the energy or teach Reiki. This is because, in the tradition of Dr. Usui, Reiki has always been handed down as oral teaching, which means that a competent energy transfer can only take place through direct contact with a living Reiki Master who has been initiated into that true lineage.

Grand Master Hawayo Takata once said, "Those who abuse Reiki will lose it," and we see the truth of this in the messages we get from people. For your own benefit, therefore, you should learn to differentiate and follow only the lineage of initiated Masters. It is important to find out how long, and from what lineage, a Master has practiced the 1st, 2nd, and Master degrees, and by whom she or he has been initiated.

A person who wants to become a Master/Teacher should have three years of experience practicing the 1st and 2nd degree, and should have an apprenticeship with a Master for about one year before being initiated as a Master/Teacher. Reiki requires individualized teaching and supervision over a longer period of time, not only for in-depth learning, but also to allow your own process of integrating the soul and mind to take place. The initiating Master/Teacher should now have about six years (previously three years) experience as a Master/Teacher and Reiki seminar leader before he/she takes on the great responsibility of guiding other students to Mastership.

We hope this advice will help you receive the gift of the *healing hands* of Reiki.

Reiki Testimonials

Testimonials by Seminar Participants

We would like to thank the participants at a Reiki seminar who reported their experiences with Reiki healing. We have selected representative responses here that we believe can be useful for those who have yet to experience Reiki.

How Did You Experience Reiki?

"It was an exciting experience that has changed my life. I can treat myself now, anytime I like."

"Beautiful. Very soothing and relaxing, a positive experience."

"I was impressed by its simplicity. I know I am acting in Divine perfection when I give Reiki, and this makes me feel calm and peaceful and gives me the courage to treat with Reiki."

What Was Your Most Special Experience?

". . . I felt my roots for the first time in my life."

". . . love."

"A very deep and intense feeling of gratitude closely connected to a feeling of happiness. I found the path to GOD again."

". . . being able to stop smoking during the seminar with Horst's help."

"I felt more at ease and carefree than I have for a long time; especially in the area of the heart, I felt pulsating energy. (I fasted during the class)."

"The fourth initation was the most special one, I felt a tremor going through my whole body."

". . . feeling my hands getting very warm, and feeling gratitude."

How Do You Feel Now (Physically, Mentally, Spiritually)?

". . . stronger and healthier."

". . . more balanced and quiet, sympathetic, loving, and ready to help others."

"Very well. I am grateful that this energy flows through my body and that I am able to pass it on to others."

"Physically I feel fit, mentally I feel cheerful, alert, and very clear, which in my case cannot be taken for granted. Spiritually I feel very harmonious, loving, and balanced."

"Simply very well. Even at work today people said I was different and was looking very well."

How Are You Experiencing Your Hands After the Reiki Initiations?

". . . more sensitive, closer to my soul. I feel in my hands a particular, pulsating life."

"My hands are warmer than usual. Even when I start giving Reiki and my hands are cold, they become warm right away."

"My hands are more sensitive and more loving in their touch."

". . . a stronger flow of energy."

Self-Healing Reactions During the Seminar

"I could release stress in a very short time."

"A migraine headache was gone within a few hours."

"Chronic cramps and stress were released."

What Is Reiki to You?"

Reiki is:

"Love in action"

"Immeasurable power"

"The opening of hearts"

"Healing and relaxing"

"Joy"

"to perceive God within me"

"A path to self-awareness"

"Love, peace, joy, courage, confidence"

"Profoundly calming"

"A great transference of energy"

"to come home"

My Path to Reiki

"Looking for a book on healing, I was browsing in a bookstore just as a young woman entered and asked about a REIKI healing book. Hearing this, I asked her what it was, and after her a short explanation of the method, I knew Reiki was what I was looking for. The bookseller then recommended an introduction lecture the next week and I attended it.

"Two weeks after this lecture, a 1st Degree Reiki Seminar was given not far from my home and I received the first Reiki initiation. I am grateful to my teachers Horst and Edith for giving me something as wonderful as Reiki, and I'll never forget how I was led to it." (*Gerda*)

* * *

"Reiki changed my life comprehensively and I am very grateful to my Reiki Master, through whom much became possible. I still have problems, but the way I handle them has changed; my contact with other human beings, everything, is more rewarding, with more intensive joy and sorrow. Reiki brought me closer to the light that is the core of everything—the closer we come to the light, the closer we come to wholeness." (*Erica*)

Experiences During Reiki Treatments

"In most cases, Reiki confronts people seemingly in a state of spiritual dormancy with facts that trigger a period of spiritual questioning. Before we had Reiki, we had a lot of colds, but now almost none." (*Nina*)

* * *

"A whiplash that had been unsuccessfully treated by doctors was healed after the man received his first Reiki treatment. Before, the man could not be without his cervical collar for longer than half an hour, but after the treatment, he didn't need it anymore." (*Walter*)

* * *

"A man arrived with an intense toothache and his face was swollen. His dentist was not available, so I gave him Reiki on his face only. After about ten minutes he breathed deeply and said he was feeling better. After a few more minutes, the pain was totally gone. The swelling lasted till evening, and there was no recurrence the next day." (*Jürgen*)

* * *

"Mrs. K., who had been taking strong medicine for years, had non-specific cramps starting in her legs and going toward her heart and head, and because of the pain, she could not lie down very well. When I gave her the first treatment, I noticed her pulse was very fast. I put one hand on the heart area, the other on the pulse, and within a few minutes her pulse normalized. Now six months have passed and the pulse is still normal. After about five or six treatments, the pain vanished; when the cramps return, which is very seldom, they are weak, and she hardly ever takes the medicine anymore." (*Siegfried*)

* * *

"An eighteen-year-old girl I treated was always tired, cold, and exhausted, with ice-cold hands and feet. She fidgeted a lot, so I had to shorten the time treating her. Her hands and feet got warm right away, and on the same day she felt much better. When I gave her the second Reiki treatment, I noticed that a warm flow of energy started at her feet and moved up through her limbs to her head. By the third treatment, I only touched her feet. After two minutes, she jumped up and said it was too hot. I never saw her again, but her mother told me she has totally changed. She feels very fit and works out now, and the cold feeling and fatigue have disappeared." (*Christa*)

* * *

"In the German Alps, we had a heavy, contagious influenza. The schools were closed, the hospitals were overcrowded, the doctors overloaded. Most of the patients had a very high fever. I too caught this flu, so I stayed in bed for a day and treated myself with Reiki. And the very next day, I was up again and rather active.

"But even as I felt better, my son Andreas had developed all the signs of this influenza, and his got worse fast. The throat was severely swollen, he had bronchitis, his fever escalated horrendously, and he was apathetic. I also had a slight recurrence and felt weak and stuffy, but decided to treat my son.

"At first I gave him Reiki in the Basic Positions, the kidneys, and the soles of his feet. After that, I lay in bed and treated myself, then sent a distant Reiki treatment to Andreas, doing this until late at night. I felt great relief and Andreas had a quiet night. Every night for a full week, I sent him a distant Reiki treatment during his sleep, and his condition improved daily.

"Before treating Andreas, I was very aware that I should not get personally involved in his treatment, but should instead be the channel for the flowing divine energy. Because I was allowed to receive and to pass on Reiki, I did not feel weakened during the treatment." (*Renate*)

Specific Treatments

"One evening my parents and my boyfriend called with complaints and accusations about me, and I could feel their negative energy dragging me down. I went to bed, but could not calm down. Then I remembered your anti-stress hand position. I started self-treating with it right away, and within ten minutes felt more balanced. I also used the color foil for cleansing and balancing the aura. I put it under my pillow and soon I was calm and could feel the Reiki energy flowing. I was happy to have this protection." (*Irene*)

* * *

"Patrizia, a fifteen-year-old girl, had an asthma attack and she cried heavily. Treating her clavicles brought immediate sedation and terminated the attack." (*Edith*)

* * *

"I treated a woman's painful wrist fracture that had plates and screws attached. I put both hands around her wrist and twenty minutes later the pain was gone." (*Jutta*)

* * *

"Reiki is very effective if a person has the sniffles. When I treated the first position on my mother's head for two minutes, it stopped her runny nose. Lymph drainage of the head completed the treatment and her sniffles never came back." (*Herta*)

* * *

"Thanks to Reiki, my breast tumor has practically disappeared, without a doctor, and without an operation. My doctor touched my breast, and shook her head, without saying a word." (*Margrit*)

* * *

"A forty-eight-year old woman had depression for years and had been treated with 460 sessions of analysis when I saw her. After giving her four Reiki treatments, her psychological blockages were released, and she is now almost healed." (*Frank*)

Testimonials of Reiki Experiences with Animals, Plants, Objects, and Technical Equipment

"In our garden, my niece found a young bird that had fallen out of his nest. He cheeped miserably, was restless, and did not want to eat. For hours the whole family had tried unsuccessfully to help him, but when I arrived, I put the bird gently in my hands and did Reiki. He calmed down at once, and after a while ravenously ate the bread given to him on a toothpick." (*Elfriede*)

* * *

"I love animals very much and they feel this. A ravishing dog named Daphne, a female setter, put her head on my lap during dinner. I petted her as often as possible, particularly her head, which had a wart in the middle of it. The owner told me her dog had this wart for a few weeks and she was planning to have it examined. Two days later, however, the wart disappeared and never returned. Daphne's owner was very happy and had no doubt that Reiki made it go away." (*Ilse*)

* * *

"An acquaintance was watering a friend's flowers. Included was a cyclamen from her recently deceased mother. This plant, particularly, was entrusted to her, and although she gave it enough water and loving care, it still wilted. Her solution was to treat the plant with her Reiki hands for about fifteen minutes, and the next day it was fresh and healthy again, and remained that way." (*Angelika*)

* * *

"During Christmas vacation my office closed for ten days. I had prepared my plants so they had enough moisture. But a *Dieffenbachia* plant fell down and all the leaves were dry when I returned to the office on the 6th of January.

"I cut the plant back and replanted it in the old pot. From my computer, I could see the plant in the window, and I treated it with Reiki for five days, sending it distant Reiki six or seven times a day, for about five minutes each time. It took about eight weeks, but today the plant has all new leaves, many of them growing from the roots, and it will again be a stately shrub.

"The other plant is a *Galactea* that came to Germany from Italy. The blossoms were dry, and when the leaves wilted all of a sudden, it looked like the plant had no more joy in life. I changed its location and treated it twice directly with Reiki (2nd degree) for about five minutes each time. For the next week, whenever I thought about it, I gave the plant short distance treatments, and after three weeks new leaves were seen and the roots were starting to sprout." (*Hannelore*)

* * *

"My situation: the headlights of my car were left on during the night, and when I attempted to start the car, there was no sound. Just as an experiment, I gave my car a distant Reiki treatment. What a joyous surprise... on the first try, the engine *purred* like a contented cat." (*Ingeborg*)

* * *

"This incident, hard to believe, will probably only be understood by Reiki friends. We had rented an apartment for our winter vacation. The caretaker was supposed to turn the heater on two days before our arrival so the house would be warm, but when we arrived, it was ice cold. There was a note on the table: 'I tried for two days to start the heater, but it does not work. Tomorrow the repairman is coming.' Outside it was ten degrees—inside not much more. My husband tried for two hours, the heater started, but the pump did not work. Just for fun I tried Reiki directly on the pump, and after a few minute, it started to gurgle. You could hear noise in the pipes, and then they slowly got warm." (*Rosemarie*)

* * *

"A few days after a 1st degree Reiki seminar, I treated a malfunction in the ignition system of my car. The cause was not clear, but ever since, it has been running. The car treatment convinced me of Reiki's powerful effect more than other physical changes I could explain in other ways, and I now feel more balanced, stronger, and less helpless." (*Nina*)

Testimonials With 2nd Degree Reiki and Distant Healing

"I would like to report on a wonderful distant treatment. In the space of a few months, my daughter hurt her eye several times, once when cutting the bushes, and another time from her baby's fingernail. The pain was enormous and painkillers did not help.

"The eye specialist said the cornea had a fissure, and he prescribed an ointment, an eye bandage, and bed rest, which was difficult for her with three little children under the age of six. To add to the problem, for no known reason her cornea burst frequently, especially under stress, heavy wind, or being in rooms where people smoked. The eye doctor warned her of the possibility that the burst would not heal and scars would remain. He recommended using a lot of the ointment, but said no other help was available. That was when I started distant Reiki treatments, and my wife and I are happy and grateful to say that our daughter's eye has not had a problem since these treatments began." (*Dieter*)

* * *

"In the fall of 1987 we joined a geological excursion. While we were walking through a stone pit, a woman stumbled and hurt her ankle. She looked pale and was in great pain. After I treated her with Reiki for about ten minutes, the pain lessened and she was able to resume walking for the rest of the excursion. As a novice in Reiki 2nd Degree I was surprised at the fast result." (*Margrit*)

* * *

"While hiking in beautiful mountain country, I sent distant Reiki to a friend for over an hour. I asked the mountains and glaciers to support me and I could feel their resonance. In the evening, I telephoned the person I had sent the distant treatment to and asked how she felt. "Since late morning I feel better than I've felt for a long time," she said. "I even called and told my friend who was going to care for me not to come by. I am happy that I feel better now." (*Günther*)

* * *

"I have been practicing 2nd degree Reiki since last November. At first I did not feel there was a great difference from the 1st Degree. I had no stronger resonance from patients until I treated a man with rheumatoid arthritis, and I would like to report on this experience.

"This seventy-five-year-old man had gout, rheumatoid arthritis, and congestive heart failure. He called around noon and said his knee joints were hurting so much every day that he had to use two canes to drag himself around his apartment. That day it was even worse. He was lying on the couch and could hardly stand up. I assured him I would come as fast as possible, but in the meantime I gave him a distant Reiki treatment. I felt powerful energy and started to sweat, but continued with my work until I had time to visit the man in the afternoon.

"I was amazed when he came to the door walking rather well and using only one cane. He told me that after our phone conversation he had felt a stabbing pain in his knee and then he fell asleep. After waking up, he found he could suddenly get up again and walk. He could hardly believe it and almost called to let me know it might not be necessary for me to come. I was very touched and thanked God from deep in my heart that I could be a channel for His power. I have continued to treat this patient and nowadays he walks the stairs—without a cane." (*Theodor*)

* * *

"The biggest help I experienced with Reiki 2nd Degree was three and a half weeks prior to my mother's death. Some days she had such unbearable pain, not even morphine helped her—but Reiki did. Every day, I sent her distant Reiki treatment, and one day I sent it a bit later and she noticed right away. The most beautiful gift for me and my family was that Reiki brought her relief from agony and made it easier for her to pass away. I was with her until her last breath and, thanks to Reiki, at the end she was breathing calmly as she released herself from her battle with cancer." (*Claudia*)

* * *

"A friend called, feeling fearful, desperate, and abandoned. She had been in the hospital for about a week due to an inflammation of the lower abdomen accompanied by a high fever, and the doctors wanted to operate on her right away. Since the hospital was far away and we had no car, we suggested a Reiki distant treatment. Although she didn't know what this was, she agreed to it at once.

"When I visited her the next day, she was free of the fever. I treated her abdomen for about an hour and gave her a little bottle of rescue remedy. The following day I called to find out how she was, and could tell by her voice that she was feeling much better. From then on, we sent her distant treatments daily.

"When the physician examined her again, he could not detect any problems. The antibiotics were stopped and she was discharged after a week." (*Hertha*)

Appendix

For Inquiries about Reiki Workshops

Brigitte Müller
Auf der Schanz 19
D 65936 Frankfurt am Main, Germany
Ph: 0049-69- 34 826 338
Website: www.brigitte-mueller.de
Email: reiki@brigitte-mueller.de

Horst H. Günther
Taunus Strasse 112
D-61381 Friedrichsdorf, Germany
Ph: 0049-6172-71887
Website: www.creamo.de
Email: info@creamo.de

For a List of International Reiki Masters

The Reiki Alliance
P.O. Box 41
Cataldo, ID 83810 USA
Website: www.reikialliance.com
Email: info@reikialliance.com

References

Bach, E. *The Bach Flower Remedies*. New Canaan, CT: Keats Publishing, 1979.

Bach, E. *Heal Thyself*. Sun Publications, 1985. http://www.bachcentre.com/centre/download/heal_thy.pdf

Bach, E. *The Twelve Healers and Other Remedies*. Sun Publications, 1988. http://www.bachcentre.com/centre/download/heal_thy.pdf

Baginski, BJ, Sharamon, S. *The Chakra Handbook*. Twin Lakes, WI: Lotus Press/Blue Dolphine, 1991.

Baginski, BJ, Sharamon, S. *Reiki, Universal Life Energy*. Mendocino, CA: Life Rhythm Publications, 1988.

Bell-Werber, E. *The Journey with the Master*. Los Angeles, CA: De Vorss and Co., 1950.

Bell-Werber, E. *In His Presence*, Los Angeles, CA: De Vorss and Co., 1946.

Bell-Werber, E. *Quiet Talks with the Master*. Los Angeles, CA: De Vorss and Co., 1936.

Blum, R. *The Book of Runes*. New York, NY: St. Martin's Press (Oracle Books), 1982.

Brown, F. *Living Reiki: Takata's Teachings*. Mendocino, CA: Life Rhythm Publications, 1992.

Burka, CF. *Clearing Crystal Consciousness*. Albuquerque, NM: Brotherhood of Life, 1986. Available as an e-book by Amazon or from website: www.clearingcrystalconsciousness.com

Burka, CF. *Pearls of Consciousness.* Albuquerque, NM: Brotherhood of Life, 1987. Available as an e-book by Amazon or from website: www.clear-ingcrystalcon sciousness.com

Cerminara, G. *Insights for the Age of Aquarius.* Wheaton, IL: Theosophical Books, Div. Quest Books, 1976.

Cerminara, G. *Many Lives, Many Loves.* Camarillo, CA: DeVorss and Co., 1981.

Cerminara, G. *Many Mansions: The Edgar Cayce Story on Reincarnation.* New York, NY: NAL/Dutton, 1988.

Diamond, J. *Life Energy.* St. Paul, MN: Paragon House, 1990.

Diamond, J. *Your Body Doesn't Lie.* New York, NY: Warner Books, 1989.

Gawain, S. *Living in the Light.* Novato, CA: New World Library, 1986.

Haberly, H. *Reiki. Hawayo Takata's Story.* Olney, MD: Archidigm Publications, 1990.

Hay, L. *Love Your Body.* Carlsbad, CA: Hay House, 1989.

Hay, L. *Heal Your Body.* Carlsbad, CA: Hay House, 1988.

Hay, L. *You Can Heal Your Life.* Carlsbad, CA: Hay House, 1987.

Jampolsky, GG. *One Person Can Make a Difference.* New York, NY: Bantam Books Publishing, 1992.

Jampolsky, GG. *Love Is the Answer.* New York, NY: Bantam Books Publishing, 1991.

Jampolsky, GG. *Out of Darkness Into the Light.* New York, NY: Bantam Books Publishing, 1989.

Jampolsky, GG. *Love is Letting Go of Fear.* Berkeley, CA: Celestial Arts Publishing Co., 1988.

Jampolsky, GG. *Goodbye to Guilt.* New York, NY: Bantam Books Publishing, 1985.

Jampolsky, GG. *Teach Only Love.* New York, NY: Bantam Books Publishing, 1984.

Kelder, P. *The Eye of Revelation: The Original Five Tibetan Rites of Rejuvenation.* Eureka, CA: Borderland Sciences Research Foundation, 1989.

Kubler-Ross, E. *On Life After Death*. Berkeley, CA: Celestial Arts Publishing Co., 1991.

Kubler-Ross, E. *Death, The Final Stage of Growth*. New York, NY: Touchstone, 1986.

Kubler-Ross, E. *Living with Death and Dying*. New York, NY: Macmillan, 1982.

Kubler-Ross, E. *On Death and Dying*. New York, NY: Macmillan, 1970.

Moody, R. *The Light Beyond*. New York, NY: Bantam Books Publishing, 1989.

Nelson, R. *Door of Everything*. Camarillo, CA: DeVorss and Co., 1963.

Price, JR. *The Abundance Book*. Carlsbad, CA: Hay House, 2005.

Price, JR. *The Planetary Commission*. The Quartus Foundation for Spiritual Research, Inc. Boerne, TX: Quartus Books, 1984. http://www.quartus.org/The PlanetaryCommission.htm

Price, JR. *Practical Spirituality*. Carlsbad, CA: Hay House, 1996.

Purce, J. *The Mystic Spiral*. New York, NY: Thames and Hudson, Inc. 1980.

Ray, S. *Inner Communion*. Berkeley, CA: Celestial Arts, 1990.

Ray, S. *Pure Joy*. Berkeley, CA: Celestial Arts, 1988.

Ray, S. *I Deserve Love*. Berkeley, CA: Celestial Arts, 1987.

Ray, S. *Drinking the Divine*. Berkeley, CA: Celestial Arts, 1984.

Ray, S. *Celebration of Breath*. Berkeley, CA: Celestial Arts, 1983.

Ray, S. *The Only Diet There Is*. Berkeley, CA: Celestial Arts, 1981.

Ray, S. *Loving Relationships*. Millbrae, CA: Celestial Arts, 1980.

Sams, J, Carson, D. *Medicine Cards*. Rochester, VT: Inner Traditions/Bear & Co., 1988.

Scheffer, M. *Bach Flower Therapy*. Rochester, VT: Inner Traditions, 1987.

Smothermon, R. *Handbook for the Third Millenium*. Santa Rosa, CA: Context Publications, 1991.

Smothermon, R. *Conversations with Life*. Santa Rosa, CA: Context Publications, 1987.

Smothermon, R. *The Man-Woman Book*. Santa Rosa, CA: Context Publications, 1985.

Smothermon, R. *Transforming Number One*. Santa Rosa, CA: Context Publications, 1982.

Smothermon, R. *Winning Through Enlightenment*. Santa Rosa, CA: Context Publications, 1980.

Yogananda, P. *Where There Is Light*. Los Angeles, CA: Self-Realization Fellowship, 1988.

Yogananda, P. *Whispers from Eternity*. Los Angeles, CA: Self-Realization Fellowship, 1986.

Yogananda, P. *How You Can Talk to God*. Los Angeles, CA: Self-Realization Fellowship, 1985.

Yogananda, P. *Songs of the Soul*. Los Angeles, CA: Self-Realization Fellowship, 1983.

Yogananda, P. *Man's Eternal Quest*. Los Angeles, CA: Self-Realization Fellowship, 1982.

Yogananda, P. *Science of Religion*. Los Angeles, CA: Self-Realization Fellowship, 1982.

Yogananda, P. *Scientific Healing Affirmations*. Los Angeles, CA: Self-Realization Fellowship, 1981.

Yogananda, P. *Autobiography of a Yogi*. Los Angeles, CA: Self-Realization Fellowship, 1981.

Yogananda, P. *Law of Success*. Los Angeles, CA: Self-Realization Fellowship, 1980.

Yogananda, P. *Cosmic Chants*. Los Angeles, CA: Self-Realization Fellowship, 1974.

Yogananda, P. *Metaphysical Meditations*. Los Angeles, CA: Self-Realization Fellowship, 1964.

INDEX

ABOUT THE AUTHORS

Brigitte Müller, the first Reiki Master/Teacher in Europe, was initiated into Reiki in Canada by Phyllis Lei Furumoto in 1983. As a pioneer, she successfully lay the the foundations for making Reiki Healing Treatments well known in Europe. Starting out in her native Germany, she attended business school, became an executive secretary, and went to England to learn English. For several years, she lived in California and later returned to Germany where she was married and divorced. The author's quest for a spiritual path during this difficult time in her life first led her to the teachings of Paramahansa Yogananda of the Self-Realization Fellowship, then, during a 1981 visit to California, she was guided to Reiki and received the 1st Degree. She knew at once this was her calling, and was so inspired that she organized the first Reiki Seminars for her Master/Teacher, Mary McFayden, in Hamburg and Frankfurt. While Mary was teaching in Germany, the author assisted in her seminars, translated for her, got her own Master training, and was initiated by Mary into the 2nd Degree. Brigitte lives in Frankfurt, Germany and teaches the traditional Usui Shiki Ryoho System of Reiki there and in many countries around the globe.

Horst Günther, born in Frankfurt, Germany, was a businessman managing a company and exploring many ways to help people when he experienced Reiki at one of Brigitte's first workshops in Germany It was clear he felt a deep connection to Reiki and ended up assisting Brigitte in her seminars as she guided him towards becoming a Reiki Master/Teacher. The course of this author's life changed dramatically when Phyllis Lei Furomoto, Carrier of the lineage of the Usui Shiki Ryoho System of Reiki, initiated him as a Reiki Master/Teacher in 1985, and later gave him her blessings to train and initiate new Reiki Masters/Teachers. When he is not leading Reiki workshops in many countries around the world, or teaching seminars in Rebirthing and Kinesiology, Horst lives and teaches in Friedrichsdorf, Germany.